The Boxer's Workout

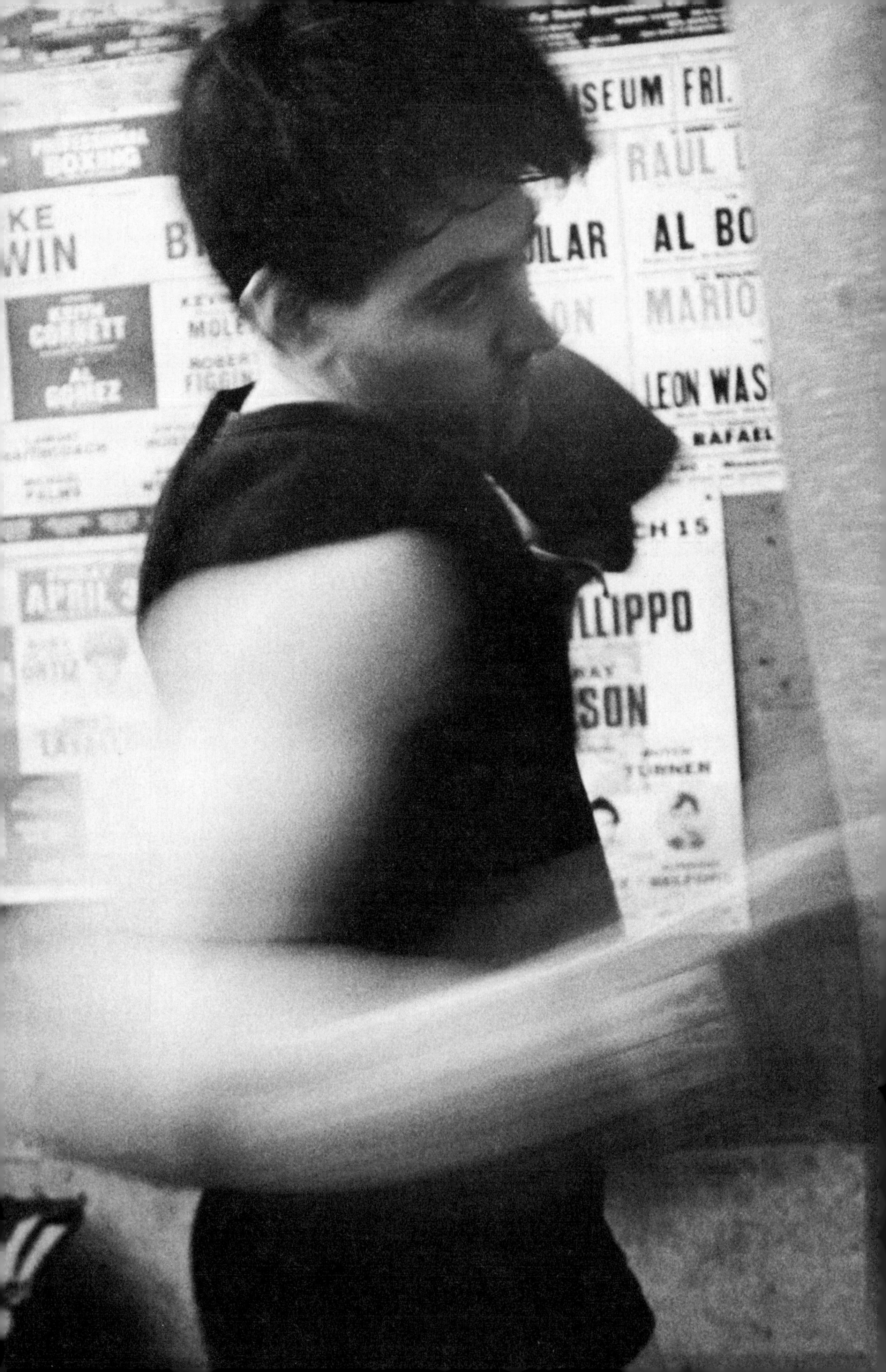
SEUM FRI.
RAUL
AL BO
ILAR
MARIO
LEON WAS
RAFAEL
BOXING
KE
WIN
CH 15
ILLIPPO
SON
TURNER

The Boxer's Workout

Peter DePasquale

FIGHTING FIT, INC.

New York
1990

FIGHTING FIT INC.
PO Box 021334
Brooklyn, NY 11202-0029

Photographs by Vincent Aiosa
Cover concept by Lenore Buonocore

Library of Congress Cataloging-in-Publication Data

DePasquale, Peter,
  The boxer's workout.

  FIGHTING FIT, INC.
  1. Exercise.   2. Boxing — Training.   I. Title.
GV461.D375   1988   613.7'044
ISBN: 0-9627050-04
Library of Congress Catalog Card Number 90-82757

FRONTISPIECE: *Actor John Haran on the heavy bag. "Let's face it. You can't punch a fitness machine."*

When you make a fist, something primal happens—a return to your roots that sets the stage for a deeper, more satisfying kind of fitness that will make you more effective in your professional life.

This book is dedicated to the growing legion of white-collar men who make a boxer's workout an important part of their professional success—to their courage, élan, and continued good fortune.

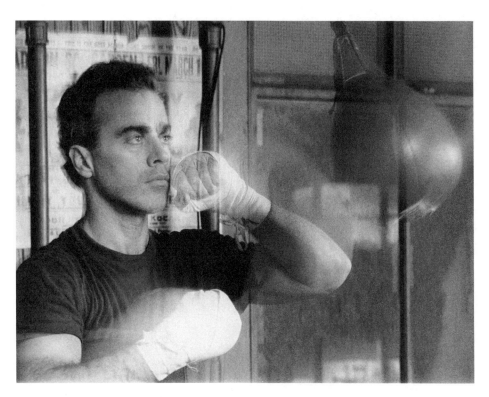

Actor/writer Joseph Carberry on the speed bag.

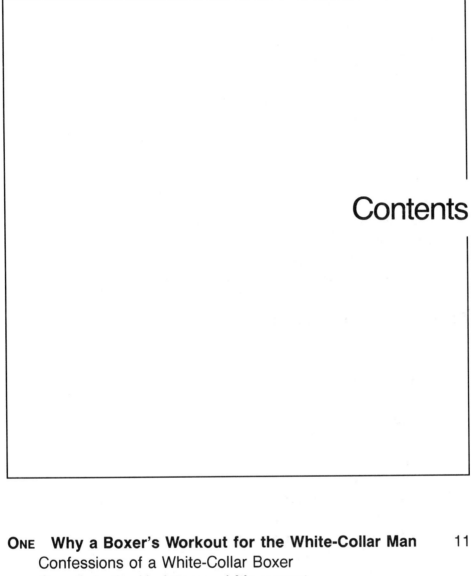

Contents

The Boxer's Workout

One

Why a Boxer's Workout for the White-Collar Man

CONFESSIONS OF A WHITE-COLLAR BOXER

Something was missing.

It had been about one year since I received my vice president's title, and my career was still going great guns, but something was missing. I began working harder and longer, hoping to fill the void. But no matter how exciting I tried to make my advertising job, how many new business pitches I got involved in, how many client presentations I made, no matter how hard I tried to bury it in my day-to-day routine, I couldn't shake the feeling in my gut. Get up, put on a suit, take the train to the office, meetings-meetings-meetings, take the train home, late supper and an hour of prime-time TV, sleep. Jogging every other morning.

It wasn't the job. I enjoyed advertising. I enjoyed the people I worked with. I even enjoyed my clients. It was more a feeling of loneliness, of detachment from something important, something exciting and at the same time grounding. I decided to return to the Gramercy Boxing Gym.

I hadn't been to the Gramercy for several years, since my amateur boxing days. I had a modest amateur boxing career, fighting no more than five or six bouts a year because schoolwork or business projects would inevitably interfere with my training and my manager wouldn't let me compete unless he felt I was absolutely prepared. While I certainly wasn't the cream of an amateur crop whose stars included Sugar Ray Leonard and Howard Davis, I remember getting a rush out of being known around the gym as "the tough college kid" and at college as "the marketing major who's a Golden Gloves boxer."

I loved boxing: stepping into another dimension every time I walked into the gym; training hard alongside the best professionals; the pure life-on-the-edge excitement of every sparring session and match. (And it was great knowing—for what it was worth—that I could dump even the most arrogant teaching assistant or computer science wiz on the seat of his pants.)

My visits to the gym became less frequent, then stopped, as I devoted myself to my advertising career. Yet I knew that it was boxing that helped me rise quickly at work. Let's face it: after you've gone toe to toe with a well-trained boxer whose objective is to make you unconscious in front of your friends and loved ones, and have survived, even the most pressured new business presentations or the most arrogant client heavy can't shake your confidence. At age twenty-seven I became one of the youngest vice presidents in the history of the second-largest advertising agency in the world, managing a $13-million budget for one of its most important clients.

Going back to the Gramercy Gym was scary. I could hear thumping, pounding sounds as I creaked up the sacred stairs of the oldest boxing gym in New York City—the same stairs that carried Floyd Patterson and José Torres, both of whom trained at the Gramercy on their way to the championship of the world. My throat tightened

12

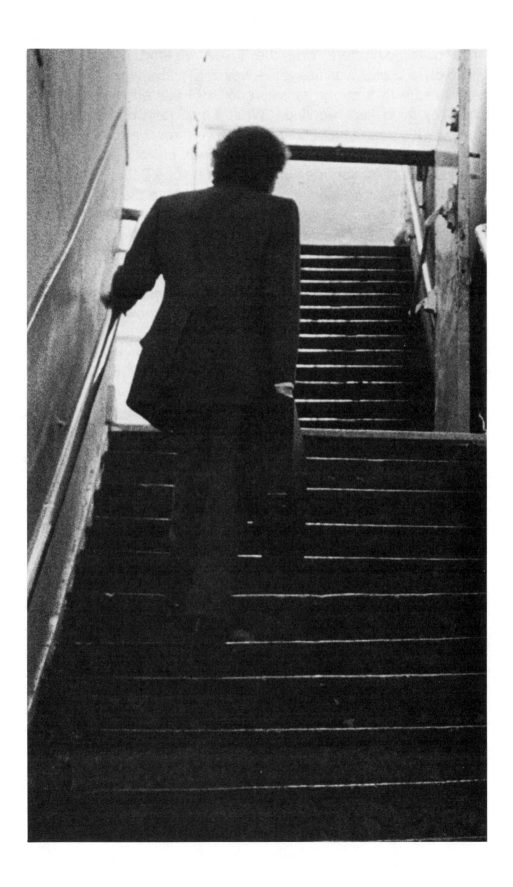

as I began doubting: "The boxers you knew are surely gone. The boxers here now will look at your suit and briefcase and wonder what you're doing here. Then they'll see you start to work out and think you're a businessman gone weird." The thumping got louder and mixed with a strong sweaty odor as I started up the second flight. My mind kept working: "What if you look bad during your workout? It's been four years since you've thrown a combination or hit a heavy bag. You're crazy. You're out of your element. You should be back at your desk, where you belong."

I felt like the new kid in class as I walked onto the crowded gym floor. Action all around me. A middleweight in a rubber suit firing combinations at the heavy bag. Lightweights shadowboxing gracefully in one ring, two clumsy heavyweights sparring in another. Trainers shouting instructions, speed bags slamming against their wooden platforms, jump ropes hissing. Effort, sweat, straining, striving. I could feel my nervousness start to lift. I knew I was where I belonged.

"Peter!" I turned and saw Al Gavin, who had been my trainer and was still a great friend. "Step into my office . . . ," he said as he gestured toward a small desk in a corner of the gym. Al Gavin and his partner Bob Jackson run the Gramercy. For over twenty years they've trained and developed many of the best amateur and professional boxers in New York City. They're two of the best men in boxing or anywhere—straight shooters who know their business. "Look, I'm not gonna tell you how to run your advertising career," Al said, "but I will tell you that it's good for you to cut loose and come down here and work the floor a few times a week. Let's see if we can find you a locker . . ."

I began doing a boxer's "floor workout" three times a week. The floor workout is a unique noncontact regimen practiced by amateur and professional fighters to build the tremendous fitness they need to succeed in both sparring and matches. The workout includes: warmup exercises and stretches; practice of the key movements and punches in front of a full-length mirror; shadowboxing in the ring; sessions on the heavy bag, speed bag, and jump rope; followed by stomach exercises. I hung a heavy bag and speed bag in my garage so I could replicate the workout at home on days when it was difficult to get to the Gramercy, and I began doing light roadwork on the days between my much harder boxer's floor workouts.

14

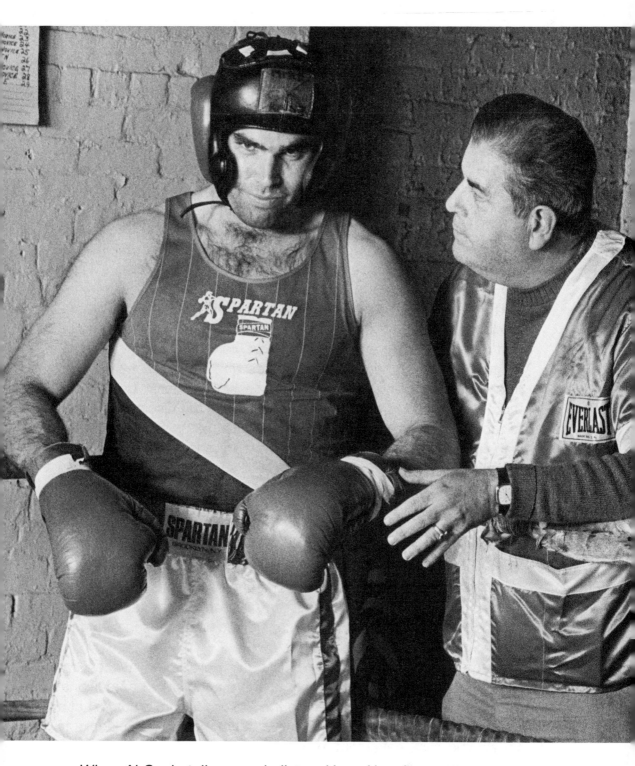

When Al Gavin talks, people listen. Here Al makes a recommendation to Martin Snow, a block of granite from Fordham University.

15

Amazing things happened. I began to feel a new vibrancy, once again tasting a fitness I hadn't known in years. I lost weight—and kept it off. While pounding the heavy bag or slamming the speed bag, I was finally able to leave the office not just physically, but fully. Working out became a spirit-refreshing release instead of a physical maintenance chore. After several months I began to complement my skill and fitness-building boxer's floor workouts with occasional sparring, under Al Gavin's supervision, against some of the growing number of white-collar men who do a boxer's workout at the Gramercy. Sheer excitement and fun. A chance to try the moves and punches I'd honed during my floor workouts against a real live opponent in an atmosphere of learning. An experience and ritual I was proud of, that became a part of me.

The tenets of effective boxing weren't left at the gym. With renewed enthusiasm, I applied these "rules of the ring" in the office and became a more effective manager: More objective evaluations of my own strengths and weaknesses and those of my account team as the starting point for a successful business battle plan; more focused objectives and work plans, and the discipline to stick to those plans; new flexibility to make adjustments when presented with unforeseen opportunities. And most important, new confidence to finally break away and start my own successful marketing and communication consultancy, fulfilling one of my greatest professional goals.

I invite you to make the Boxer's Workout an exciting new part of your professional regimen. I've put together this handbook with the help of Al Gavin, Bob Jackson, and the white-collar boxers of the Gramercy Gym. It brings you the workout professional boxers use to get fighting fit. While the focus is on the noncontact floor workout routine, discussion of controlled, supervised sparring is included for those who wish to go further.

Many of the photographs in this book were taken at the Gramercy, to bring you the unique atmosphere and spirit of a traditional boxing gym. However, you can do the Boxer's Workout not just at a serious boxing gym like the Gramercy, but at most fitness clubs or in your home gym, basement, or garage.

The book is written from my white-collar practitioner's point of view. It is straightforward and no-nonsense—just like the workout—

and is sensitive to your lifestyle and schedule. It assumes no prior experience with the art of boxing—just your heartfelt desire to break out from under the fluorescent office lights. Start doing the Boxer's Workout now. You'll gain new fitness and confidence. You'll have more fun than you've ever had since college. And you'll discover you're not alone. . . .

GROWTH IN THE UNDERGROUND MOVEMENT

There is a remarkable upsurge in white-collar boxing. From accountants to actors, from writers to brokers, from doctors to entrepreneurs—more white-collar men than ever before fit a boxer's workout into their day. Some seek out the environment of a serious boxing gym like the Gramercy. Others train at their local YMCA or fitness club. Still others enjoy the solitary release that comes with slamming a heavy bag in the privacy of their own garage. Why are these men turning to boxing?

Kevin McCloskey, a thirty-four-year-old art-packaging foreman for a fine arts company, enjoys the individual challenge. "I've always tested myself physically and mentally, but I've found nothing that compares to boxing. Unlike team sports, there's no one but yourself to blame for failure. For demanding total concentration, look no further."

Ray Ginther, a thirty-five-year-old sales director for a leading publishing concern, is attracted by the physical benefits. "It's a total workout that builds upper body, legs, quickness, endurance, strength, timing, and overall toughness. It requires very little special equipment and provides a competitive challenge."

The confidence-building aspect is an important ingredient for Alan Caminiti, communications manager for Control Data Corporation. "Boxing is a microcosm of life, and what you do in the gym can be extrapolated to life. Are you willing to take risks? Move in? Boxing gives you confidence in everything you do, a willingness to make the tough decisions."

George Haywood, a bond trader at Shearson Lehman, who learned to box at Harvard, points out the strong similarity between boxing and his business. "Trading is a lot like boxing. You have to beat the other guy to the punch. It's a second-to-second thing. You have to be real quick, nimble, and keep your wits about you. You have to like competition and not like losing. The more successful traders are pretty competitive people—they don't like to lose."

THE PHYSICAL BENEFITS

The boxer needs it all: power, speed, endurance, reaction, flexibility, and balance. His workout routine of stretching, shadowboxing, heavy bag, speed bag, jump rope, stomach exercises, complemented by roadwork or other aerobic exercise (swimming, bicycling), gives him the unique whole-body conditioning his sport demands. His legs, hips, back, shoulders, arms, and midsection are all worked hard as they're trained to work together. He builds aerobic fitness *and* muscular strength, develops power *and* balance, quickness *and* stamina. Then he puts it all together in one lean, efficient fighting machine. Joseph Russo, a twenty-five-year-old draftsman/designer, puts it simply, "You use muscles you haven't used in years —or ever, for some people."

A Boxer's Workout helps build a healthy heart. You get all the cardiovascular benefits of whole-body strength and endurance training: improved circulation to the extremities, greater stroke volume, lower resting pulse, quicker recovery times. And perhaps even more important, a Boxer's Workout gives the unique stress reduction that only comes with hitting something. What could be healthier than letting go of anxiety and anger in an appropriate way? "Let's face it," says John Haran, a twenty-five-year-old actor, "you can't punch a fitness machine."

A Boxer's Workout burns fat and builds muscle. And it helps you *keep* weight off, since the excitement of the workout makes you want to do it more consistently.

MENTAL TOUGHNESS

Boxing toughens your mind. Tom Carrillo, a thirty-five-year-old free-lance producer/writer, cites the wisdom of the late Cus

18

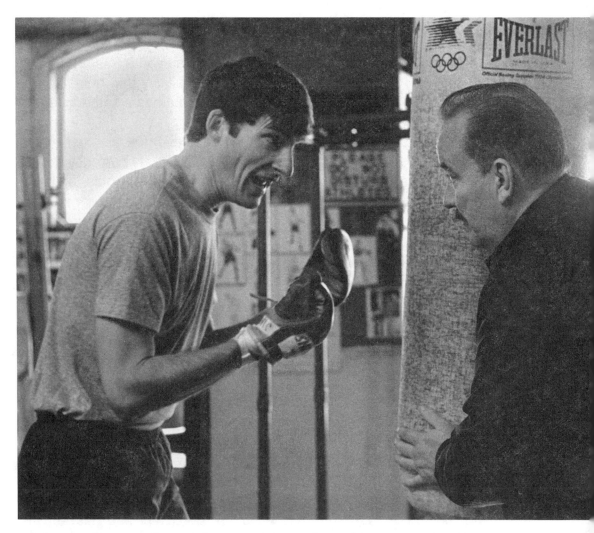

James Grant, editor of Grant's Interest Rate Observer, *a leading financial publication, checks technique with Bob Jackson.*

Damato. (Damato trained champions Floyd Patterson and José Torres, and was the trainer and dominant force in the development of Mike Tyson.) "Cus Damato said it best when he said that boxing teaches you to overcome fear. He didn't mean that boxing would take away fear completely, but that it would teach you to live and function well within that fear."

The mental toughness aspect is an important reason Oliver (Jim) Sterling turned to boxing. Sterling is the founder of Sterling Drilling and Production, a large natural gas development company. He won the New York Athletic Club's light-heavyweight championship in 1982. "Boxing sharpens your senses. It gives you a forward-driving attitude, a healthy aggressiveness and sensitivity that helps you to seize the opportunity in business. The workout has a cathartic effect that leaves you in a better frame of mind."

"No doubt about it, the mind is the key to eventual success in this sport," says Michael Groves, a twenty-five-year-old currency trader. "The intensity level is high. There are no excuses, no ifs. I am the bottom line. The end is a level of movement and skill that is complex, fast, and mentally very demanding."

THE WORKOUT THAT THRILLS—AND MORE

Madison Square Garden. You're fighting for the heavyweight championship of the world. The bell rings to start the fifteenth round. You leave your corner and confront Muhammad Ali a final time . . .

Own up. We've all dreamed of that golden moment when we've dumped Ali on the seat of his pants. Or stopped Marciano right in his tracks. A Boxer's Workout lets you live that moment as often as you like. It brings you a character, a mystique, and a dream that you can't get from the most rigorous aerobics class or the highest-tech exercise machines. It puts you in that special, exciting place that's unique to the manly art. "Working on the heavy bag has left me feeling exhilarated," says Steven Silverstein, a forty-year-old mental health administrator at a leading metropolitan psychiatric center.

As if the physical, mental, and excitement benefits of a boxer's workout aren't enough, there's more—

The Only Workout for the Older Man

No pampering. No coddling or lightened-up senior-citizens' calisthenic routines. Just exciting new fitness from the sport you've loved since you were a kid. Dr. Howard Miller, a seventy-year-old surgeon, does a Boxer's Workout regularly at the Gramercy. "I wanted to enter a whole new world—a physical world—and see

20

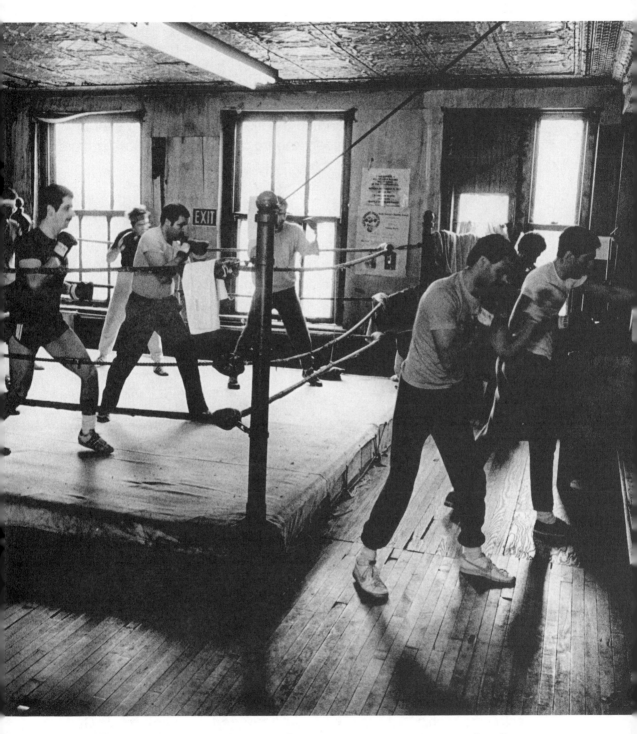

White-collar boxers during a Saturday morning class at the Gra-mercy.

what it was like," he says. "I wanted to stick my nose (not my chin) in," he adds with a smile. The result: "Most of the guys have forgotten my age. The happiest part is that I'm beginning to forget it, too." Dr. Miller, currently working on a book about the nature of the human thought process, also cites the mental aspects: "The greatest courage I've shown is walking up the stairs to the gym—it's a formidable flight when one considers the boxers at the top. Boxing gave me the chance to conquer fear and panic."

The Burgeoning Network

There's a special bond among white-collar men who practice the manly art. You'll feel it the moment you extend your hand to that new marketing director or project manager and say, "I do a Boxer's Workout, too." And you'll feel it throughout the life of your relationship—a mutual, unspoken identification and trust that permeates your interactions.

Adaptable and Portable

The Boxer's Workout is easily adapted to meet your individual schedule. "The workout is something I can do at home with a minimum of equipment and hassle," says John Nodtvedt, a computer systems consultant. "Some sports require great expenditures, club fees, travel, and waiting on line. This I can do in my own home gym."

The Boxer's Workout travels well. A modified version keeps company president/boxer Jim Sterling fit on his frequent business trips. "I just move around some furniture in my hotel room, and do my shadowboxing, jump rope, and stomach exercises. It takes me very little time, and I feel great."

A Rich History of Civilized Participants

"If necessity obliges a man to be a blackguard, he may as well be scientific," opined Lord Byron, who sparred frequently with Gentleman John Jackson, the heavyweight champion of the day.

Boxing is a sport of choice for the civilized man. The attendees at

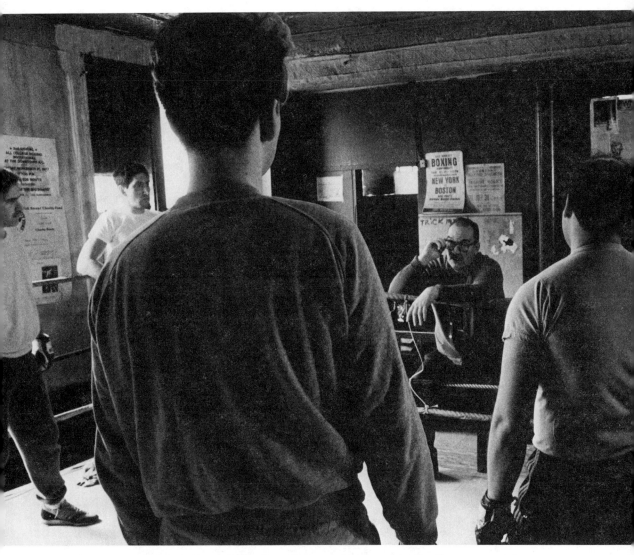

Bob Jackson instructs his charges in the same Gramercy ring where champions Floyd Patterson and José Torres honed their skills.

virtually any major bout during virtually any era include a *Who's Who* from the worlds of business, politics, literature, and entertainment. What's more, many of these men have themselves climbed into the squared circle; for fitness, competition, or both.

Alumni from the business world include J. Paul Getty, who sparred frequently with Jack Dempsey; and Bernard F. Gimbel, a

23

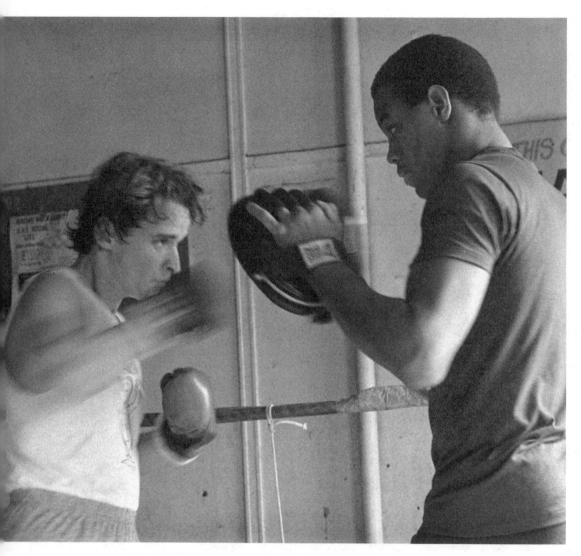

Kevin McCloskey, art-packaging foreman for a fine arts company, shoots a right toward a mitt held by Tyrone Howard, a professional actor and a white-collar boxing instructor.

sparmate of Gene Tunney; and Alfred I. DuPont, who became a lifelong friend of John L. Sullivan after engaging the ''Boston Strong Boy'' during an all-comers challenge at a burlesque house. A long list of statesmen is headed by Theodore Roosevelt and ranges from George Wallace to Gerry Brown, with Gerald Ford bringing us back toward center. Men of letters include Ernest Hemingway (who if he

24

were alive would probably insist on being listed first), George Bernard Shaw, Budd Schulberg, A. J. Liebling, Jack London, and of course Norman Mailer. And the world of entertainment gives us Miles Davis, Eddie Murphy, Billy Joel, Tony Danza (who was a promising professional boxer before he turned to acting), John Huston, Ryan O'Neal, and Mickey Rourke.

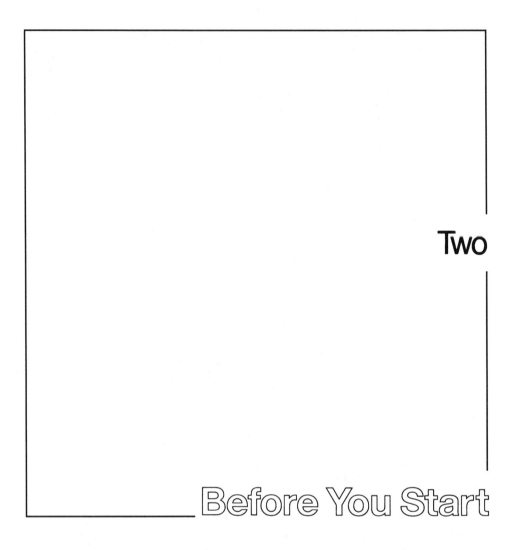

Two

Before You Start

PRECONDITIONING

The Boxer's Workout is strenuous. Ease into it gradually by establishing a preconditioning period. During this time you'll develop an aerobic fitness base and get your mind and muscles used to the essential physical moves of the sport.

The preconditioning period should be about a month, depending on your current physical condition and on how quickly you take to the key boxing moves described in Chapter Three. What should preconditioning include? Follow the action plan below.

Consult your physician before beginning this or any other fitness program.

Begin light roadwork to establish an aerobic fitness base. Review the purpose and method of roadwork, which are described separately on pages 29–32. During your preconditioning period, do roadwork every other day, then every day. Use roadwork to build your aerobic fitness to a point where you can easily run a mile within ten minutes. Your ten-minute mile should be run conventionally, at a steady speed, without any of the shadowboxing/pauses which are so much a part of the roadwork that helped get you into shape in the first place.

It should be noted here that while roadwork is the quintessential complement to a boxer's workout and in the character and spirit of the sport, swimming, bicycling, or rigorous walking ("fitness walking") are perfectly acceptable substitutes for the white-collar boxer. These activities are also aerobic in nature and are easier on the joints—an important consideration if foot strike aggravates that nagging knee injury that's a permanent reminder of high school gridiron glory. If you choose swimming, bicycling, or fitness walking as a roadwork substitute, be sure to set and achieve a performance goal that you believe indicates a base level of aerobic fitness in line with the ten-minute mile.

Practice the essential physical moves of boxing, which are described in Chapter Three. To maximize the physical benefits, enjoyment, and safety of the Boxer's Workout routine, it is recommended that you first get familiar with the basic physical moves of the sport. Rehearse each of these punches and movements in front of a full-length, wall-mountable mirror. (These are available for about ten dollars at any mass-merchandise or housewares store.) Perform each move in slow-motion and work up to a moderate speed. Don't punch too hard—your back and shoulder muscles aren't ready yet. Practice these moves during short sessions throughout your preconditioning period, until they begin to feel comfortable. You'll notice that in addition to building your working knowledge of boxing mechanics, each practice session provides mild exercise in itself; enhancing your base fitness level.

When you can comfortably run a ten-minute mile (or have met a comparable base aerobic fitness goal and are comfortable with boxing's key punches and moves, you are physically ready to begin the Boxer's Workout (Chapter Four). Once you start doing the Boxer's Workout, your roadwork/bicycling/swimming should be done only every other day—its purpose at that point is to provide an important "easy day" workout between much harder "Boxer's Workout" days. (More on the importance of a "hard day–easy day" approach later in this chapter.)

To Precondition Mentally

Recognize that a gradual approach is the best approach. Serious amateur and professional boxers vary the intensity of their training in accordance with their fight schedule. They train hardest during the weeks immediately prior to a match, pushing their fitness level right up to that point where they are as strong as they can possibly be, but where only a small amount of additional intensive training results in fatigue, sluggishness, or even sickness. Sometimes, they go over that edge—witness the many cases of the fighter who looks great in training camp yet performs sluggishly and without inspiration during his match. "I just couldn't get my punches off—I didn't feel right" is the typical postfight lament.

Professional fighters and their managers constantly confront this fine line between optimal fitness and overtraining. As a white-collar boxer, you don't (and shouldn't) have to. For you, boxing is an ongoing fitness program. While a boxer's workout enables you to taste the excitement of the sport, the fact is that you *don't* have a big-money fight coming up. So train gradually and at a moderate level. Don't overtrain—it's not healthy and it's not necessary.

Recognize that progress might not be linear, and might not be immediately apparent. You'll inevitably run into periods when it seems like you're not improving. Work through them. For some boxers (the author included), progress seems to come in uneven spurts rather than in steady increments. Patience. Just about when you're flagellating yourself most severely, you'll have that "breakthrough" workout when, suddenly and surprisingly, everything comes together.

28

Relax. Boxing calls for the smooth, efficient execution of technique. From Sugar Ray Robinson to Muhammad Ali to Roberto Duran to Marvelous Marvin Hagler, the best boxers are relaxed. If you feel yourself rushing or tightening up, simply pause and take a few deep breaths of that wonderful commodity called air; then slowly begin again—relaxed.

ROADWORK

Roadwork is important for four reasons:

It is the cornerstone of your preconditioning program, providing the aerobic fitness base which is essential to safely complete and enjoy the Boxer's Workout.

Once you begin the Boxer's Workout, it provides the important "easy day" portion of the hard (Boxer's Workout) day–easy day approach recommended for the white-collar boxer. Specifically, it provides the enhanced circulation which delivers greater amounts of oxygen and nutrients to muscles stressed during the prior day's Boxer's Workout, and helps remove waste materials left in those muscles.

The easy run-and-box/pause-and-box nature of roadwork will get you still more comfortable with boxing's key physical moves.

From a mental standpoint, roadwork is a vital component of the boxing experience. It gets you feeling like a boxer.

How to Do It

Roadwork isn't all-out running. It's not a plodding jog either. It's a one- to two-mile light, springy run of varying but moderate speeds, interspersed with light punching and periods of shadowboxing. Run, punch and run, stop and shadowbox, run again. Run faster, slower; straight and zig-zag. The mood is upbeat. You control the action. When you've finished, you should feel energized—not exhausted.

While professional boxers do roadwork every day, the white-collar practitioner need hit the road only every other day; between successive Boxer's Workout days. Although it's called "roadwork,"

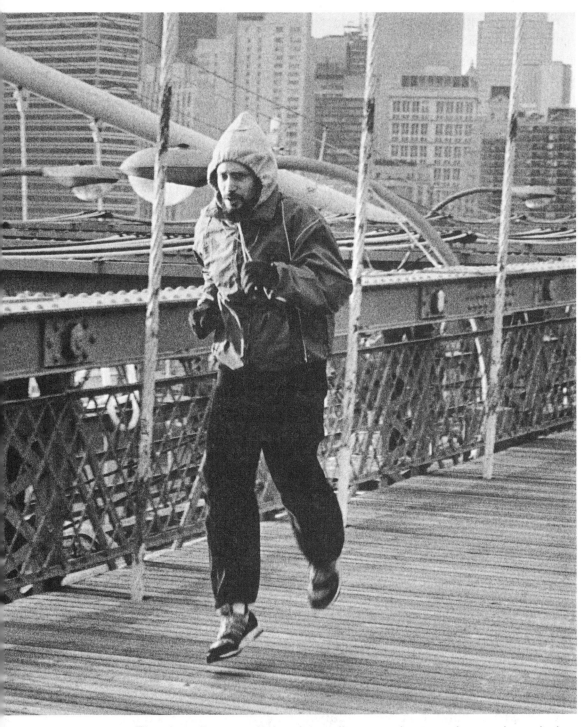

The loneliness of the long-distance boxer: the author during roadwork on the Brooklyn Bridge.

you should favor softer surfaces, if possible, because they're easier on the joints.

Don't run too fast, or too far. Remember—roadwork constitutes the "easy day" portion of your program, when your stressed muscles rest and rebuild. If you overdo it, it will have precisely the opposite effect, increasing the risk of injury and leaving you more stale than week-old bread. "I left my fight on the road" is a common complaint of overtrained boxers.

If possible, do roadwork in the morning. The air is cleaner—it's a fresh, new day. During summer you beat the heat. During winter the cold, cutting air wakes you up with the invigorating rush that professional boxers from Tunney to Tyson have come to know and love. The aforementioned circulation enhancement and its benefits take place earlier—there's less soreness to carry around the rest of the day. There's more privacy, fewer people to yell "Rocky" at you. And when you're done, you feel "cleaned out," physically and mentally, and ready to take on the world. So get out of bed early and do it—it's worth it.

Dress right. This is tricky at first, since your speed and intensity (and thus how warm you feel) vary during the roadwork session. By trial and error you'll eventually learn just what to wear during any given time of year. Until then, err on the warm side—you want to finish with a light sweat. Clothing should be loose, to allow for movement. A baggy top. Sweatpants. Wear running shoes if you have them—if not, sneakers are fine. No boots—they look great on professional boxers and marines, but this is your "easy" day. Light colors for maximum visibility. This is especially important during dark winter mornings. (Consider the reflective vests and striping that are available in most running stores.) A towel around the neck is perfect—it absorbs perspiration, provides warmth, and breathes at the same time.

Quick and easy. The session should take no more than thirty minutes from start to finish. Easy stretching, then begin roadwork slowly; the idea is to get loose as you run. Although the pace varies, try to crescendo toward the middle of the session. Walk the last hundred yards and breathe deeply. You should be breathing just about normally by the time you're back home. Get right into a warm shower so you don't chill. No calisthenics—these are part of the

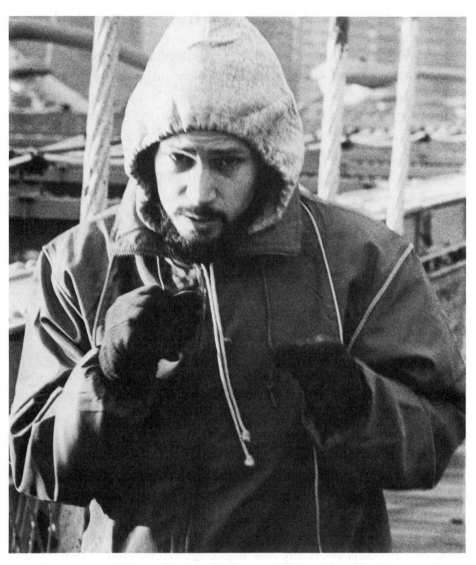

Pause periodically during your roadwork session to shadowbox.

Boxer's Workout that you do on "hard" days. Besides, you've got to get to work.

DIET AND WEIGHT CONTROL

There is significant change going on within the boxing world regarding the nature of the ideal diet. Generally speaking, the traditional ultra-high protein "steak for breakfast" approach has given way to (1) a healthy recognition of the importance of complex carbohydrates and dietary fiber, (2) greater consideration of the individual boxer's food likes and dislikes, and (3) consideration of the individual boxer's personal metabolic rate, and variances within that rate at different stages of fitness.

As a white-collar boxer, try to factor these considerations into your own approach to food. If weight is a problem, consult your doctor (or a nutritionist your doctor recommends) to develop a balanced, healthy, regular eating plan—one that's right for your unique metabolism, tastes in food, and professional lifestyle. Stay away from fad diets—the kind you "go on."

Because these diets are meant to have mass appeal, they can't precisely consider the significant metabolic rate differences from individual to individual. Further, they can't precisely consider metabolic rate changes for a specific individual as he begins and continues with a program of regular exercise.

Given healthy regular eating habits, there are two ways the Boxer's Workout can help you to control your weight:

It burns significant amounts of calories. Exactly how many varies with individual metabolism, and with the intensity and duration of "your" Boxer's Workout. During your first twelve weeks, for example, it is recommended that fewer and/or abbreviated "rounds" be completed on each exercise as you proceed through the workout. The calorie burn at this stage will differ from what you experience later, when you'll have "grown into" longer, more intensive rounds. (Beginning, moderate, and intensive Boxer's Workout levels are presented in Chapter Four.) Eventually, by regularly monitoring your weight and developing a boxer's uniquely sensitive "feel" for poundage, you'll gain a very accurate idea of how well the workout, at its various "effort" levels, burns weight for you.

It makes you more sensitive to what you put into your body. A hard Boxer's Workout session leaves you feeling "cleaned out." Progressive workouts get you leaner, sharper, and stronger—like a boxer in training. Once you experience this fitness level and feeling, you'll want to keep it. Your attitudes toward food will change. You'll want only good fuel to go into your "good" body. That's not to say

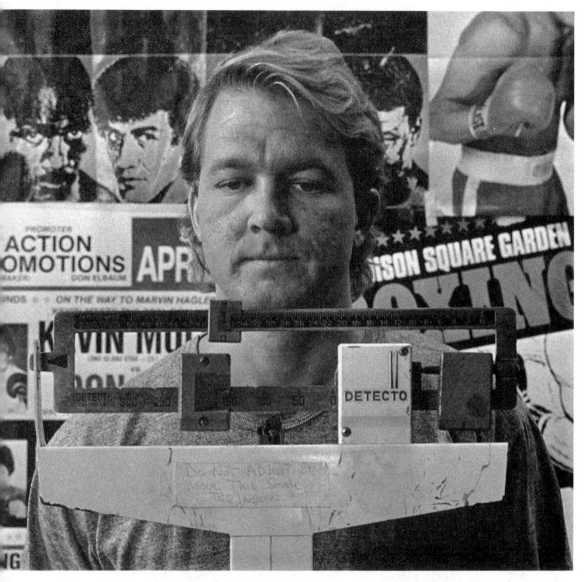

W. Gregg Porter, Assistant Dean for Administration at the Graduate School of Management at the New School, weighs in.

you'll order a steamed vegetable platter at your client's favorite steakhouse, or a Moussy when pitching a prospect over drinks. But you will find yourself practicing moderation—one cocktail instead of two, a fish entrée instead of beef in béarnaise sauce, fruit for dessert instead of cheesecake. And should you occasionally "overdo" it, don't worry; with regular Boxer's Workouts and healthy everyday eating habits, it won't show up on the scale.

Beyond what we've covered, use your judgment. You know the basic food groups. You know that as Americans we tend to overconsume animal proteins and fats, sugar and sodium, and that we take in way too much cholesterol. You know when you're eating right and when you're eating wrong—for you. And that the business lunch, with all its temptation, is an important part of the way that business is done. So use moderation and control, but don't beat yourself up on those occasions when you "overdo it."

MY PERSONAL EATING HABITS

My diet is essentially vegetarian. It includes pasta, whole-grain bread and cereals, beans, brown rice, and plenty of leafy vegetables, complemented by eggs and occasionally some fish. While it might seem very "unboxer-like," I've learned through trial and error that this diet is just right for me: it gives me the relatively greater amount of complex carbohydrates I feel I need for rigorous Boxer's Workout sessions. It provides the amino acids I need to rebuild muscle tissue, without any or all of the cholesterol, fat, growth-stimulant residues, and dyes which are commonly found in meat. It's light on my system and easy to digest. (I hated the groggy, "heavy" feeling which seemed to come over me after I ate meat.) Further, it makes business lunches light and easy—almost every restaurant (steakhouses included) offers a healthy selection of salads, pasta, and fish. And it tastes great. (As a third-generation Italian-American, I'll take pasta any time.)

Two final notes before we leave this area:

Drink water—before, during, and after your workouts. Dehydration is cause for poor performance and is dangerous. What's more, it sneaks up on you. Good runners, for example, know that thirst is not a good indicator of the body's need for water—the feeling of thirst comes too late, after you may have already dehydrated to a degree that will adversely affect your performance. A water jug is required equipment for the Boxer's Workout and is every bit as important as your hand wraps and striking mitts. Hydrate before every workout (drink at least a pint of water) and take a moderate

35

amount of water at least every two rounds. On especially warm days, drink a small amount after every round.

Caution: You may have heard about "drying out," the prefight water-deprivation process that professional fighters sometimes undergo in order to make a weight classification limit. Forget it. The better fighters and trainers know that drying out is unfortunate and dangerous—unfortunate because it indicates a lack of careful weight control during training, and dangerous because it saps a fighter of vital body fluids at the very time he needs them most. "Drying out" has no place in the Boxer's Workout or in recreational boxing.

Monitor your weight at regular intervals. Not too frequently— the daily fluctuations, or lack of them, can be discouraging. Not too occasionally either, since you'll want to be aware of a significant trend in either direction before it's too far along. Every three or four days is fine. Weigh in at about the same time of day every time. Again, don't overreact to a change one way or the other. You're looking for slow, safe, healthy weight loss or weight maintenance.

WHEN AND WHERE TO TRAIN

Frequency

For maximum benefit, the Boxer's Workout should be done three times per week, with (lighter) roadwork on "off" days. A prototype schedule which reflects this "hard day/easy day" approach might include Boxer's Workout sessions on Monday, Wednesday, and Friday; roadwork sessions on Tuesday, Thursday, and Saturday; and complete rest on Sunday. Budget from forty to seventy minutes for each Boxer's Workout session, depending on your fitness level and the workout intensity you desire. (Beginning, moderate, and intensive Boxer's Workout levels are discussed in Chapter Four.) Budget thirty minutes for each roadwork session.

THE IMPORTANCE OF A "HARD/EASY" APPROACH

Stress followed by rest equals improved performance. As athletes, we all too often focus only on the first half of this equation.

Spurred on by the work ethic which is so much a part of us, we train, overtrain, and injure. Then, after allowing barely enough time for our injuries to heal, we rush back into intensive training as if we had never missed a day—only to suffer injury once more.

Recognizing this tendency toward overtraining and injury, a growing number of exercise physiologists and sports medicine experts, as well as leading boxing coaches, are urging us to take a "hard/easy" approach to training, one which gives equal consideration to the "rest" portion of the stress-rest equation. To more fully explain the importance of rest, a simple yet important description of the physiological dynamics of rigorous fitness training appears below. It captures in layman's terms the essence of what the experts have described and verified through carefully controlled studies. From my own humble standpoint as an athlete driven to improve, I believe the experts are right. I've suffered often as a result of the overtraining-injury cycle they warn against; I've literally "felt" what they describe clinically.

DURING A HARD WORKOUT

- Your muscle fibers get stressed, a portion of muscle membrane gets "torn down," and cell membranes get broken and twisted.
- Your glycogen stores get depleted. Glycogen is the fuel stored in your muscles—it combines with oxygen from the blood to power your muscles.
- Waste products, especially lactic acid, are produced as a result of the oxygen-glycogen combination.

DURING REST

Blood brings oxygen and nutrients to the stressed muscles, with the following results:

- Muscle cells are rebuilt stronger, to handle greater stress next time.
- Glycogen stores are replenished—the muscles get a new supply of fuel.
- Lactic acid residue is flushed away.

The important point is that muscles get stronger during rest, not work. Overtraining denies them this vital rest. Without time to re-

37

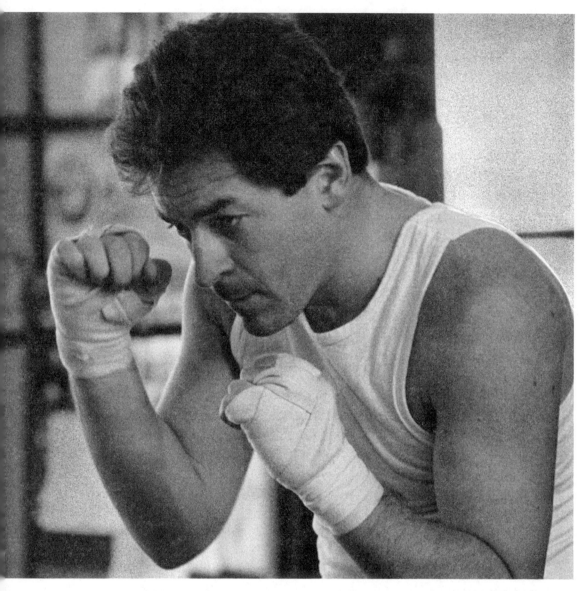

Ray Ginther, sales director for a major publishing concern: "It's a total workout . . ."

store and regenerate, they become damaged, stiff, and prone to injury. By following the recommended "hard day/easy day" approach, you'll maximize improvement and diminish the risk of injury.

Some additional notes on training frequency and the value of the hard/easy approach:

As mentioned earlier, light roadwork on "easy" days speeds recovery because it boosts circulation to stressed muscles, facilitating the "rest" benefits described above. However, use caution; if you overdo your roadwork, you will have turned an "easy" day into another "hard" day, putting new wear and tear on muscles that need rest.

The hard/easy approach, perhaps surprisingly, is in keeping with the training methods of many professional boxers. Although these pros train in the gym every day, they vary the intensity of their gym workouts to ensure adequate recovery between hard sessions. (The pros are generally in such great shape that their "easy" day appears quite rigorous to the beginning boxer. To the professional it is an easy day nonetheless.)

The hard/easy approach saves time, an important consideration for the white-collar professional. Again, you've selected a boxer's workout as an ongoing fitness program. You're not a professional boxer; there's no reason to spend countless hours in a gym as if you were.

Finally, strive to maintain a workout schedule that's as regular as possible, given the sometimes unforeseen demands of your job. Within the hard/easy approach, regularly scheduled workouts will optimize fitness, learning, and enjoyment. (The excitement of the Boxer's Workout should help here, since it makes exercise something you won't want to miss.) At the same time, don't worry if you do miss a workout or two because things are a bit too busy at the job. Remember, you're in this for the long term—one or two workouts won't make or break you. And if you've been working out fairly regularly, the extra rest won't hurt.

Location

The Boxer's Workout can be done at home, at a fitness club, or at a serious boxing gym like the Gramercy. Choose the location, or combination of locations, that best fits your schedule and provides the atmosphere you desire. Some cases in point:

- Suburban vice president who does the Boxer's Workout at home three evenings per week and never goes to a serious boxing gym.

- Time-efficient account executive who does the Boxer's Workout at his midtown fitness club during lunch hour.
- Professional writer, who does the Boxer's Workout at the Gramercy, and complements the Workout with periodic sparring.
- Senior editor who does the Boxer's Workout at home but tries to get to a serious boxing gym at least once every other week, for "an infusion of atmosphere."

There are special considerations to be made in selecting your workout environment, whether it is at home, at a fitness club, or at a boxing gym.

WORKING OUT AT HOME

The advantages here are time and privacy. Since home is where you start and end your day, you eliminate the time and trouble of a separate trip to a fitness club or gym. Privacy is a two-edged sword, however. Enjoy it for the unique feeling and atmosphere that come with working out alone—not because it protects you from "looking bad" as you learn alongside other boxers. (Fear of "looking bad" is, in my opinion, the beginning boxer's single greatest deterrent to learning. More on this on pages 69–70.)

In addition to adequate space, working out at home requires the purchase and installation of extra equipment, specifically a heavy bag, and a speed bag/platform assembly. These are available at most sporting goods stores. A good heavy bag costs under one hundred dollars, as does a good speed bag/platform. (Equipment is discussed separately, on pages 54–65.)

Finally, don't spar at home. For many white-collar boxers, the noncontact Boxer's Workout done alone and at home provides more than enough fitness, character, and enjoyment. However, you might eventually wish to try sparring. This should be done only in a serious boxing gymnasium or under controlled conditions in a fitness club, under the supervision of your trainer, and while wearing proper protective equipment. Treat sparring with the respect it deserves. Even if you regularly do your noncontact Boxer's Workouts at home, make a special trip to the gym to do your sparring. Instead of dangerously whaling away at your next-door neighbor under unsafe conditions in your basement or garage, take him with you to

40

the gym. You'll spar instead of "fight." You'll be much safer. And you'll learn much more.

The better boxing gyms provide four major benefits:

A traditional boxing atmosphere. For better and worse, there's nothing like walking into a real boxing gym. It brings out the fighter in all of us. The poster-lined walls and smell of sweat give you a sense of the tradition that underlies the unique sport in which you've chosen to participate.

The company of other boxers. Although boxing is among the most individual of endeavors, you'll quickly realize that in a boxing gym you are an individual among counterparts, each trying his best to sharpen his boxing skills. Although boxers are generally not the cheerleading type, they appreciate effort no matter what the proficiency level. There's high mileage in the occasional quiet acknowledgment you might receive from a crusty trainer or a professional boxer—not to mention the more regular support of other beginners.

Supervised instruction—if you'd like it. This book includes the essential character, moves, and workout routine of boxing. If you have the desire, time, and to some extent the money for supervised instruction, you can find it at a serious boxing gym.

Broadly speaking, there are two kinds of instruction you might consider. The first is enrollment in the growing number of boxing classes being offered by serious boxing gyms. The second entails regular private sessions with a qualified trainer. (There are several important considerations in choosing a trainer—they are discussed on pages 48–54.)

The opportunity to observe and take part in sparring. Again, you might eventually wish to go beyond the noncontact Boxer's Workout routine and take part in sparring. A serious boxing gym is the place to do this, under the careful supervision of a qualified trainer. Further, there is much to learn by carefully observing the sparring sessions of other boxers in the gym, even if you do not choose to spar.

As for negatives, there are two (related) drawbacks associated with training in a serious boxing gym: proximity and time. Since the

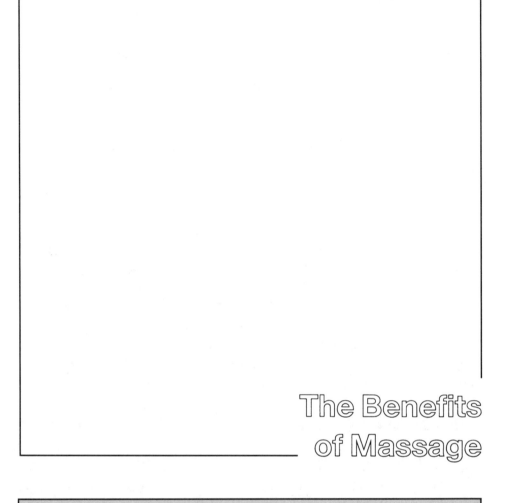

The Benefits of Massage

For years, professional boxers have made massage a part of their regimen. If possible, you should consider it too. By enhancing circulation to stressed muscles, massage speeds the restoration process and with it the occurrence of the important physiological "rest" benefits described earlier.

The two most common kinds of massage are Swedish and Shiatsu: Swedish massage has historically been more popular in the Western world, and the traditional boxing massage is Swedish in nature. Swedish massage entails a stroking and kneading of the muscles. Oil is applied to minimize friction.

(The old-time masseurs took great pride in developing their own special oils and liniments.)

Although Shiatsu is still relatively new in the West (and therefore new to most Western boxers), I recommend that you give it a try. Shiatsu, which literally means "finger pressure," is based on principles of Oriental medicine which have proven tried and true for thousands of years. In Shiatsu the practitioner applies gentle but firm pressure to various energy pathways (meridians) which run along the body. By stimulating the meridians, the practitioner helps the receiver to balance his energy. The receiver is left feeling relaxed and "centered." (More on the importance of "center awareness" in Chapter Three.)

It's relatively easy to find a massage practitioner. If you work out in a serious boxing gym, ask your trainer or the gym owner. (Many gyms have a massage practitioner on the premises during certain hours.) If you work out in a fitness club, a massage practitioner goes with the territory—all you need to do is make an appointment. If you work out at home, you might call a boxing gym or local fitness club and ask for a referral. Additionally, you might seek information at a local health-food store—they typically sell newspapers and periodicals which list local massage practitioners (for example, *Whole Life* magazine, *East-West Journal,* etc.). Ask the store owner or workers to recommend someone.

Rates vary. A full one-hour treatment (of either Swedish or Shiatsu) starts at about thirty dollars; a shorter treatment will cost less. Some massage practitioners give a lower rate per treatment if you commit to a series of treatments.

1976 Olympics—and the renewed interest in boxing that Sugar Ray Leonard and company generated there—the number and quality of serious boxing gyms located in suburban areas has grown. However, the majority of serious boxing gyms are still to be found only in large cities—and not always in the poshest sections. For the white-collar boxer, working out in a serious boxing gym might mean a separate trip to a destination not easily "on the way" to office or home. To some white-collar boxers (the author included), the separate excursion is part of what makes the boxing experience special. To others, it is simply time-consuming. An alternative: regular Boxer's Workouts at home or at a conveniently located fitness club, "spiced up" with occasional Boxer's Workouts at a serious boxing gym.

WHAT TO LOOK FOR IN CHOOSING A BOXING GYM

Some key considerations are listed below. Use them to help decide whether a serious boxing gym is the right workout environment for you, and to help evaluate one gym versus another.

What is the "tone" or feeling you get when you walk into the gym? The atmosphere in the better gyms is exactly like that of a well-run business—efficient yet comfortable. Very little talking, lots of concentration, as each boxer goes about his work.

Do successful professional boxers work out there? The pros bring an ideal no-nonsense attitude to their workouts, and this attitude permeates the gym.

Does the owner or supervisor seem to have the activity under control? And given the inherent cynicism of boxing people, is he at the same time reasonably easy for you to approach? (That is, can you go up to him and say, "Hi, I'm interested in training here, and I'd like to ask you a few questions," etc.)

Does the gym show any special orientation or inclination toward the white-collar boxer? Does it include a significant number of white-collar boxers among its membership? Does it offer classes for the white-collar boxer?

Does the gym have qualified trainers on hand to provide individual instruction should you desire it?

Does the gym have a policy toward sparring? This is important. The better gyms allow boxers to spar only under the supervision of their trainers, and they insist that each trainer control his boxer during sparring, so that a sparring session doesn't turn into a "war."

Beyond these specifics, use the overall judgment that guides you in evaluating any potential business relationship. Don't neglect your "gut feel" for the gymnasium and its people.

44

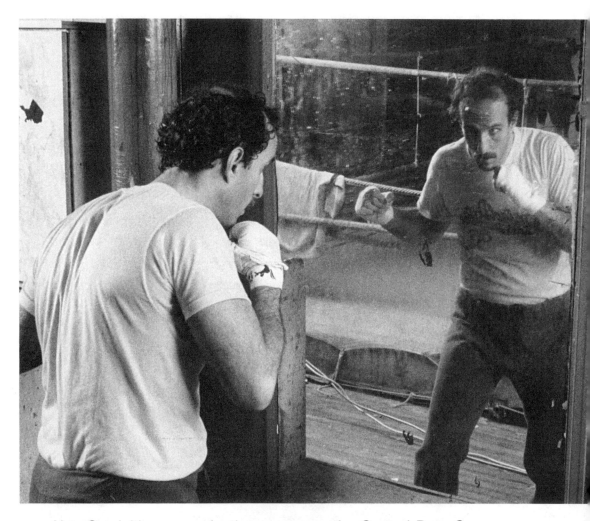

Alan Caminiti, communications manager for Control Data Corporation: "Boxing gives you confidence in everything you do, a willingness to make the tough decisions."

WORKING OUT AT A FITNESS CLUB

Generally speaking, the fitness club environment splits the difference between home and the serious boxing gym. It's "just right" for many white-collar boxers: easier to get to than a serious boxing gym, yet with more boxing "flavor" than their home workout area. A growing number of fitness clubs have recognized these advantages, and have expanded both the personnel and facilities dedicated to boxing. Many have hired licensed trainers or ex-boxers, at least on a part-time basis, to instruct beginners. Many now have a boxing "room" that houses the heavy bags and speed bags which are fundamental to the Boxer's Workout.

Some (potentially negative) factors you should consider in evaluating and selecting a fitness club:

Price. Fitness clubs are generally expensive. Although the sales representative or instructor who shows you around is quick to point

Joseph Egan, president of Capitol Marketing, a large New Jersey insurance agency, enters the solitary world of the squared circle.

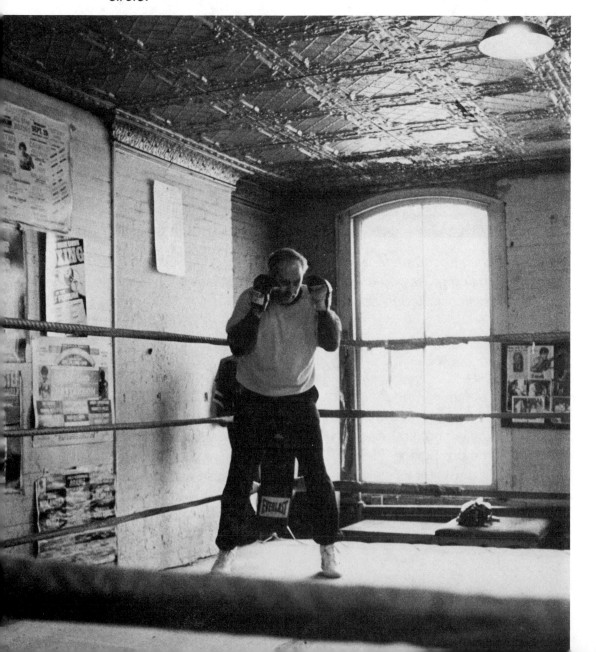

out that when you divide the membership fee by the number of days you'll use the club each year, it costs "only a couple of dollars a day," the out-of-pocket amount is nevertheless high—usually greater than the amount required to join a serious boxing gym.

Pressure. Unfortunately, some fitness clubs, especially those owned by chains, still use what many consumers describe as "high pressure" sales tactics. Make it clear to whomever is showing you around that you plan to evaluate several clubs before making a decision.

Lack of sparring. Except for the very few fitness clubs which have a boxing ring on premises, there's virtually no real "sparring" available in this workout environment. Again, while the noncontact Boxer's Workout routine alone provides sufficient exercise and enjoyment for many white-collar boxers, you might wish to spar occasionally or simply to observe other boxers as they spar. A serious boxing gym is the best place for this. While a boxing skills class at a fitness club might offer you the opportunity to "move around" at half speed with your instructor or a classmate in a makeshift "ring," which usually consists of a wrestling mat, you won't—and shouldn't —do the more serious sparring that takes place in a real boxing ring at a serious boxing gym.

Caution: Don't spar, even at half speed, without headgear, mouthpiece, and a protective cup and don't spar on a hard surface—for example, a gymnasium floor. There's always the chance, however minimal, that your partner will "overdo" it—headgear and a cushioned floor surface provide important protection from injury.

A refreshing alternative to high-priced, high-pressure fitness clubs: the good old YMCA. Despite their "old-fashioned" image, many YMCA's have significantly upgraded their "physical plant" in recent years. Further, the YMCA was among the first "fitness centers" to recognize the growth in white-collar boxing. Many local Y's are well equipped for the Boxer's Workout, offering the previously mentioned "boxing room" and group boxing instruction by qualified trainers. Their membership fees are generally reasonable, their sales approach even-handed. For these reasons a growing number of white-collar men, including Boxer's Workout practitioners, make a regular trip to the Y.

In a nutshell, choose the fitness club workout environment because it provides the previously discussed "middle ground" between home and a serious boxing gym. Don't select a fitness club, at least not exclusively, if you're interested in observing or partaking in sparring on a regular basis.

ON CHOOSING A TRAINER

If you have the desire and time to go beyond the noncontact Boxer's Workout routine and the basic boxing skills which are the focus of this book, and especially if you desire to spar, you need a qualified trainer. Once you choose to go this route, the capability and temperament of the trainer you select and the quality of your relationship will be major determinants of how good you get at the game. Before you select a trainer, gather as many relevant facts as possible, evaluate them objectively, and (again) don't neglect your "gut feel."

What to Look For

Experience. This is determined by (1) a license from the American Boxing Federation or your State Athletic Commission, and (2) a proven track record as a trainer of successful amateur and/or professional boxers. Experience in training white-collar boxers is helpful, though not critical.

Temperament. Boxing trainers are somewhat cynical, due to the character (and characters) of their game. Given that congeniality is not their forte, the more effective trainers are nevertheless approachable. In addition to readily telling you about themselves, they'll want to know a bit about what *you* wish to get out of boxing. In this way, they can design a training program that's right for you.

Time. A trainer's impressive credentials and easy temperament are negated if he doesn't have the time to instruct you. Although the better trainers are generally busier because they attract a greater number of aspiring boxers, your trainer should make the time to meet with you on a mutually agreed-upon regular basis—at least once a week.

A willingness to let you observe a training session before

you make your decision. The better trainers have nothing to hide. Without any hesitation at all, they'll invite you (or easily agree if you ask them) to let you quietly observe as they train their charges. This is something you should do before making a decision. Look for

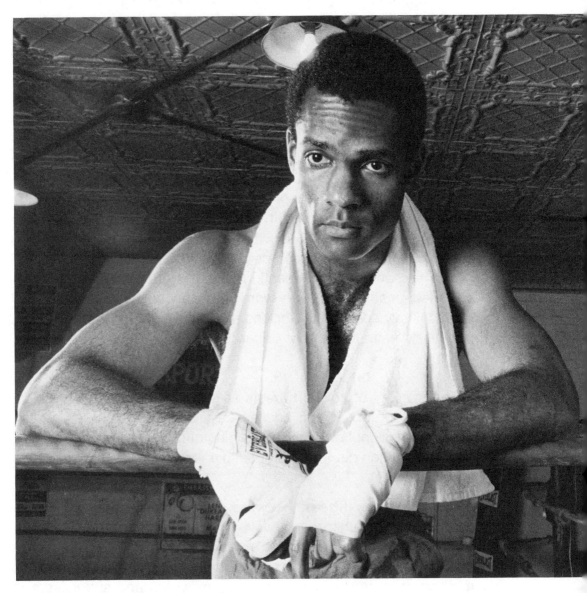

George Haywood, a bond trader at Shearson Lehman, who learned to box at Harvard: "Trading is a lot like boxing. You have to beat the other guy to the punch."

clear, quiet communication between the trainer and his boxers. The better trainer doesn't yell, scold, or condescend—he simply teaches, with great care.

An orientation toward safety. The better trainer never "throws his fighter into the ring." He works with his student slowly. Only after months of "floor work" does he let his boxer begin sparring. He picks sparring partners carefully and oversees sparring sessions closely, to maximize his boxer's learning and minimize the risk of injury.

A respect for your wallet. It is reasonable that white-collar boxers should pay more for their instruction than boxers with professional aspirations. In fact, good trainers regularly work with promising amateurs and professionals for nothing or next to nothing on an ongoing dollars-for-time basis. The trainer knows that he will be fairly rewarded through his percentage of the boxer's earnings if the boxer (due in large part to the quality of his training) becomes a contender or champion. The white-collar boxer offers the trainer no such future reward for time spent now. As a result, the trainer deserves reasonable compensation on a straight money-for-time basis. "Reasonable" is the key word here. Unless a trainer strikes you as absolutely spectacular for one reason or another, twenty dollars per session should be your upper limit.

SOME NOTES OF CAUTION

The majority of boxing trainers are good, competent professionals who work long, hard, and ethically at their craft. Like virtually every profession, however, the training of boxers has problems and "things to watch out for." Potential pitfalls are delineated below, for your protection:

Al Gavin says it best: "Beware of the towel-carriers." Towel-carriers are the unlicensed, self-appointed "trainers" who simply put a towel around their neck and do a poor imitation of Burgess Meredith in *Rocky.* They hang around serious boxing gyms like mold, despite the best efforts of gym owners and supervisors to keep them away.

The typical towel-carrier scrapes along via odd jobs and small loans from people who feel sorry for him, until he comes across an unwitting victim who "wants to learn to box." He usually meets his

50

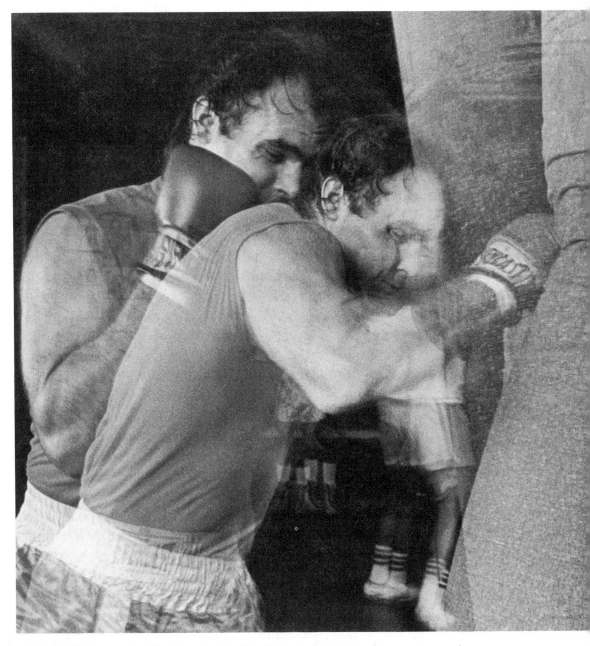

16. *You'll swear it hits back: Martin Snow during a rigorous session on the heavy bag.*

victim "on the outside," then lures him to the gym with promises of money and glory. What transpires during subsequent training (a case of the blind leading the blind) would make great comedy if it weren't so tragic for the aspiring fighter. A few of the towel-carriers boxed a little, a long time ago. Or maybe they had an uncle who was a "contenduh." Either way, they've convinced themselves that they are indisputably qualified to teach boxing. At first, I felt sorry for them, for their poor economic condition, etc. But my sympathy has evaporated over the years, as I've watched individual towel-carriers literally worm their way into a young fighter's life, and then get the fighter hurt due to their greed and/or ignorance.

As a white-collar boxer, your intelligence and lack of professional boxing aspirations (and therefore professional boxing earning potential) make you less attractive to the towel-carrier than the naive young man who "wants to make it big in boxing." At the same time, be careful—the towel-carriers can be awfully nice, even charming. When you walk into a serious boxing gym, don't talk to just anybody. Ask for the owner or the man in charge. Tell him you're a white-collar boxer interested in safe, enjoyable recreational boxing, and that you're interested in supervised instruction with a licensed trainer.

A successful fighter does not necessarily make a successful trainer. Sometimes professional boxing experience makes a man a better trainer, more sensitive to how readily his boxers can digest information, more empathetic. But sometimes professional boxing experience has the opposite effect: (1) It can cause the trainer to lose patience quickly should his student not grasp information or physical moves as readily as his teacher did; (2) it can result in the "cloning" syndrome, where the trainer tries to mold his boxer into a stylistic copy of himself during his boxing days, whether it's appropriate for the boxer or not; and (3) it can result in the trainer trying to relive his competitive boxing success through his students. This puts tremendous pressure on the beginning boxer.

The important point again: A successful fighter does not necessarily make a successful trainer. The former involves doing; the latter calls for clear, patient, sensitive teaching. Not recognizing this important distinction, a handful of ex-professionals not licensed as trainers present themselves as if they were: "I fought the best," each says proudly, "No one can teach you better than I can." But they're selling apples when you might be better served with oranges —that is, someone who's trained the best.

Beware of grandiose promises. "I'll have you moving like those guys in six months time," says the spider to the fly, as experienced amateurs and professionals work out in the background. Watch out for these kinds of grandiose promises. The better trainers simply don't make them. They know that every boxer is an individual, with his own strengths, weaknesses, and learning curve. They know that they can't possibly predict with accuracy the rate at which you'll improve until they've worked with you for at least several weeks. And even then they won't make promises about your rate of improvement. As discussed earlier, they know that progress isn't always linear. Be content in knowing that, timetables aside, a good trainer helps to bring out the best in you as quickly as it can be brought out—even if it takes a long time.

Beware of premature sparring. Again, the better trainers approach sparring cautiously. They protect their fighters. They know that "gym wars" and the resultant injuries have no place whatsoever in recreational boxing. If a potential trainer brags about how quickly he "puts his boxers in there," walk away.

WHAT DO YOU OWE YOUR TRAINER?

Honesty at all times regarding your physical condition. Be upfront about your physical condition, both before you start regular boxing training and any time during your program. As stated earlier, you should begin regular training only after sufficient preconditioning —you'll need to be in reasonable shape simply to have a productive session with your trainer. Most important, *always* communicate your condition as you approach a sparring session. If you don't feel right, haven't been working out regularly, have been sick, etc., your trainer is entitled to know so that he can take appropriate action. (He'll either postpone the sparring session or make sure it's sufficiently "toned down" to match your stamina level.)

Commitment. Before you begin supervised sessions, you should have discussed and reached agreement with your trainer on a level of commitment and frequency. Your trainer has the right to expect your regular attendance at supervised training sessions, your regular performance of roadwork on "easy" days; and your regular practice (on your own) of the moves he teaches you during supervised sessions, so that he can help you to reach your stated boxing goals.

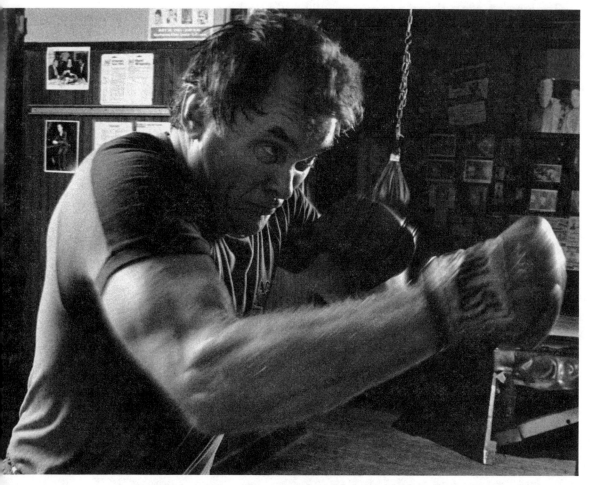

Fifty-year-old Jim Sterling, founder of Sterling Drilling and Production, throws a right that's half his age. "Boxing sharpens your senses."

Given your professional responsibilities, your trainer will certainly understand an occasional missed class or lapse in regular training. But try to minimize these—nobody likes to be taken for granted.

TOOLS OF THE TRADE: EQUIPMENT

Good boxing equipment is easy and available at a reasonable price. You can buy it at better sporting goods stores and mass-

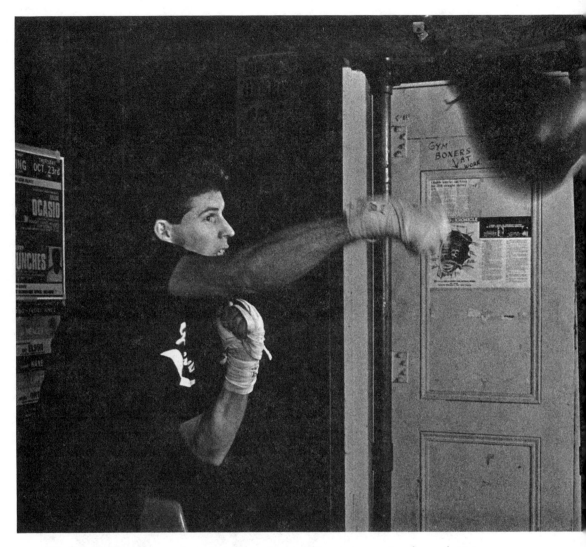

Michael Groves, a twenty-five-year-old currency trader, slams the speed bag with a flourish.

merchandise outlets. It can also be purchased through independent suppliers who make regular sales calls on serious boxing gyms. Independent suppliers are mentioned here because the author has found that the equipment they offer is usually of fine quality yet priced somewhat lower than at sporting goods stores. If you're anywhere near a serious boxing gym, ask the owner about purchasing your equipment from the supplier who calls on him. You'll save a few dollars if you have the extra time.

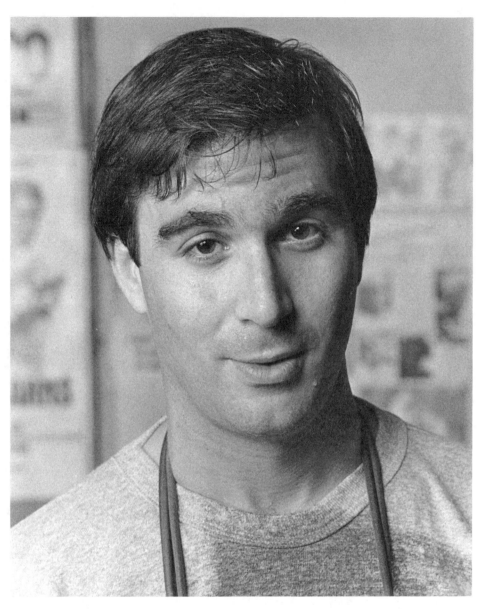

Ira Lieberman, marketing manager for a major food company, after a brisk session on the jump rope.

Buy good equipment. It generally works better, lasts longer, and provides greater protection. It's inexpensive relative to those important benefits, and compared to fitness machines and equipment required for many other sports. What's more, if for any reason you have a change of heart and decide that the Boxer's Workout isn't right for you, better equipment is much easier to sell to other boxers.

The equipment you'll need is listed below. Each item is then discussed separately. Beyond the "basic" items which are required regardless of where you do the Boxer's Workout or whether you spar, additional equipment is needed to set up for the Boxer's Workout at home, and in order to safely spar in a serious boxing gym. You can get a sense of the major items of equipment "in action" simply by leafing through the photographs in this book.

Item	Approx. Price
BASIC EQUIPMENT	
Hand wraps	$5
Striking mitts	$25–$35
Jump rope	$12–$15
Speed bag	$35–$60
Plastic water bottle	$3–$5
Boxing boots (recommended)	$25–$50
ADDITIONAL EQUIPMENT FOR BOXER'S WORKOUTS AT HOME	
Heavy bag and suspension assembly	$80–100
Speedbag/platform	$50–$85
3/4 length wall-mountable mirror	$10
Small exercise mat (for stomach exercises)	$15
Double-end bag (optional)	$40–$70
Medicine ball (optional)	$30–$60
ADDITIONAL EQUIPMENT FOR SPARRING	
Boxing gloves	$35–$60
Protective headgear	$40–$45
Mouthpiece (boil-and-mold type)	$5
Boxer's protective cup	$45 and up

Basic Equipment

Hand wraps. These are the reusable protective bandages that boxers wear to protect knuckles from abrasion and to provide a measure of wrist support. Psychologically (and to some extent physically), they merge your wrist and fist into one "unit." This is important, because it minimizes the chance of wrist injury that can occur if you bend your wrist as you land a punch. To encourage this thinking and feeling, hand wraps are worn throughout the Boxer's Workout, even when you're not actually striking the heavy bag or speed bag. (The hand-wrapping process is described and photo-illustrated on pages 65–67.)

While the majority of boxers use standard cotton hand wraps, some (including the author) prefer elastic (Ace) bandages instead—because they provide a "tighter" wrap without cutting circulation, and because the end of the bandage is easily "tucked" back into the bandage itself. (Standard hand wraps need to be "tied," which can be difficult if there's no one around to do it for you.)

A pair of hand wraps costs about five dollars, give or take a few cents.

Striking mitts. Striking mitts, also called "bag gloves," are the "smaller" gloves worn when hitting the heavy bag. Some boxers also wear them while hitting the speed bag. When selecting striking mitts, look for (1) plenty of padding, to better protect your knuckles; (2) lots of space on the inside, so you won't have to struggle to fit your wrapped hands into the mitts, and (3) a leather rather than vinyl shell, for greater durability and protection. Don't buy poorly constructed striking mitts; knuckle abrasions are painful. A good pair of striking mitts costs $25–$35.

Jump rope. Buy a leather jump rope with ball bearings built into the handles. Ball-bearing handles are a must in order for the rope to move quickly. Similarly, stay away from ropes made of cotton fiber —they "flop" when you try to jump rapidly. Finally, don't use a "plastic" rope—the kind where a thin cotton rope is covered by tiny plastic cylinders of assorted colors. The rope inside the cylinders can wear out without your realizing it. Suddenly millions of colored cylinders scatter across the gymnasium floor, and you self-consciously apologize to the pros as you pick up each piece individually. You can invest in a good leather jump rope with ball-bearing handles for twelve to fifteen dollars.

Speed bag. Some gyms or fitness clubs provide speed bags. They simply leave the bags up all day, for whoever wants to use them. In the majority of cases, however, you'll need your own speed bag. (It's better to have your own anyway, since you can select the one that's just right for you.)

Again, stay away from vinyl. The bag should be made of leather, with an inflatable bladder inside. The "loop" at the top of the bag clips into an attached ball-bearing swivel. When you want to work on the speed bag at a serious boxing gym, you simply screw your speed bag into the platform provided.

The smaller the bag, the faster it moves, with "peanut"-type speed bags moving the fastest. Start with a larger bag and get your timing and technique right. As you improve, you'll "move down" to the smaller bags.

A good speed bag ranges from thirty-five to sixty dollars in price. A smaller bag usually costs more than a larger one. This is because smaller bags are made tougher—to absorb the greater beating they necessarily take per square inch of surface.

Plastic water bottle. As discussed previously, take small amounts of water frequently during your workouts. A one-quart plastic water bottle with a screw-off cap is perfect. Some boxers use the squirt-top plastic bottles that bicycle riders use. (I find that if I'm really thirsty, it takes forever to get sufficient water through the squirt top.) And then there's the tried-and-true method the old-time trainers use: Take an old whiskey bottle, wrap it with several layers of medical tape to protect against breakage, and write your name on it.

Boxing boots. These are optional but recommended. If you plan to stick with the Boxer's Workout, buy them. They give greater ankle support than sneakers, and they provide traction without "sticking" to the canvas ring floor or the hardwood gymnasium floor the way sneakers do. They're also lighter than most sneakers. The better you get at boxing, the less comfortable you'll feel in sneakers.

Boxing boots are available in nylon, leather, and in nylon-and-leather combinations. The author has used all three kinds with satisfaction. Nylon boots give sufficient ankle support and feel lighter on the feet. Leather boots seem to give greater ankle support than nylon and seem to last longer.

Boxing boots range in price from twenty-five to fifty dollars. Leather boots are usually closer to the upper limit.

Heavy bag and suspension assembly. While you're hitting the heavy bag, it might seem unfazed by even your most powerful punches. But over time the bag really does take a beating. So buy a good one.

Heavy bags have either a canvas or nylon surface. Both surfaces work about equally well and cost about the same. As for poundage, heavy bags are available at forty- and seventy-pound weights. A forty-pound bag is of course easier to handle when you hang it in your garage or home fitness area, and is cheaper (although not by an amount commensurate with its lower weight). While the forty-pound bag works fine, a seventy-pound bag is recommended if you can accommodate it—the extra poundage will help you to develop greater punching power. Expect to pay about sixty-five dollars for a forty-pound bag, about eighty dollars for a seventy-pound bag.

The bag is suspended by a hook-and-chain assembly. You can construct the assembly easily and economically with a visit to your local hardware store. The assembly starts with three or four light-weight chains of equal length (the exact number varies depending on the number of ring supports built into your bag). The chains emanate separately from the top of the bag and join at the end of a heavier chain, which is in turn hooked to the ceiling or a beam. You can expect to pick up the lightweight chains, the heavier chain, the ring that connects them, and a ceiling hook—all for about twenty dollars. This puts the total cost of your heavy bag and suspension assembly at approximately eighty to one hundred dollars.

Speed bag/platform. This circular platform is easily wall-mount-able. Consider only "solid" wooden platforms, as these are sturdy, enable the bag to move rapidly, allow you to vary the size of the bag that you screw in, and minimize vibration against your wall. Stay away from "hollow" metal rim-type platforms. They confine you to only one bag size and fall short in each of the remaining areas. Expect to pay from fifty to eighty-five dollars for a good speed bag platform.

3/4-length wall-mountable mirror. This is available at any hardware, houseware, or mass merchandise outlet. It should cost about ten dollars, and it goes up easily.

Small exercise mat (for stomach exercises). Also dubbed a "personal fitness mat," "personal exercise mat," etc., these are made of a thin layer of foam covered with vinyl. They are available at any sporting goods store for no more than about fifteen dollars. A (cheaper) piece of plain foam works just as well, if you have one around or can get one easily.

Medicine ball (optional). You won't need this right away, but when you've reached a point where you can easily do the basic stomach exercises (sit-ups and crunch) described in Chapter Four, consider making this investment. Medicine balls range in size and price, from about thirty dollars for a four-pound ball to about sixty dollars for a fifteen-pound ball. The heavier you are, the heavier the ball you want: I weigh one-hundred and forty-five pounds and am more than challenged by a nine-pound ball, which cost me forty dollars.

Double-end bag (optional). This apparatus should really be called the double-end *ball,* because the central component is a leather or hard rubber ball, about the size of a soccer ball. The ball rests at eye level, suspended by an elastic rope which emanates from the top of the ball and is fastened to the ceiling and a corresponding rope which emanates from the bottom of the ball and is fastened to the floor. When you strike the ball, it of course goes in the direction of your punch, then quickly swings back toward you with about equal force. The idea is to slip the ball the same way you might slip a punch, and then "time" the ball so that your next punch strikes it flush. The tighter you rig the supporting ropes, the faster the ball goes.

The double-end bag is up and is available at most boxing gyms. It is optional equipment if you do the Boxer's Workout at home. In any event, you don't need this item right away. You'll first want to practice and get comfortable with slipping without anything "coming at" you. (The ball can make quite an impression if you don't slip quickly enough.) When you feel you're ready, you might work the double-end bag into your Boxer's Workout routine.

A leather double-end bag costs about sixty-five dollars, a rubber bag about thirty-five dollars. In this case you might consider buying the cheaper bag, because the bag itself doesn't take all that much of a beating (compared to a speed bag, for example). Add five dollars for hooks to fasten the support ropes to the floor and ceiling

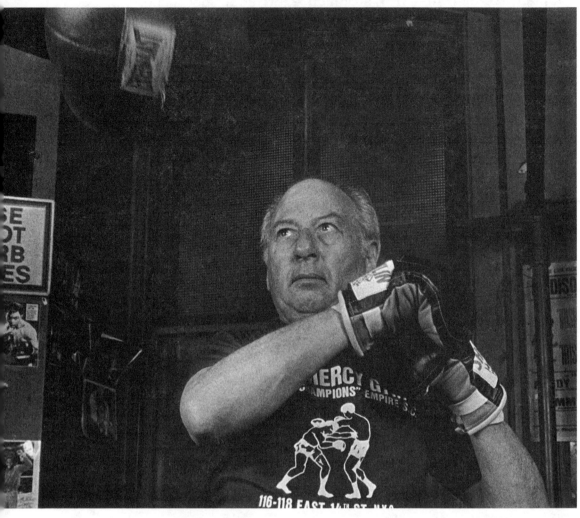

Dr. Howard Miller, a seventy-year-old surgeon, on the speed bag, "I wanted to enter a whole new world—a physical world—and see what it was like."

(pick up the hooks at your hardware store) and we're talking forty to seventy dollars altogether.

Additional Equipment for Sparring

This equipment will be needed if you wish to spar in a boxing gym.

Boxing gloves. A good pair of leather boxing gloves are as personal to their owner as a baseball mitt to a ballplayer. Over time you "break them in" so they're just right for you. (Uncomfortable or unfamiliar gloves are the last thing you'll want on your mind as you head out of your corner to spar.) So buy only top-quality gloves. And don't lend them out. (The better fighters recognize the "personal" nature of equipment, especially gloves. They buy their own, and rarely lend or borrow.)

Fourteen-ounce gloves are commonly used by boxers in all weight classes up to light-heavyweight. If you weigh over 175 pounds, buy sixteen-ounce gloves. The price ranges from thirty-five to sixty dollars.

Protective headgear. Headgear is available in several different styles and sizes, each affording a different degree of protection. The rule of thumb is that "more is better." More protective padding is better than less; a model with built-in "cheek protectors" is better than one without. The better models offer this extra protection without compromising your range of vision. A good headgear might feel cumbersome or uncomfortable when you first try it on in the store. Stick with it—you'll gradually get used to it, and in the long run you're of course better off with the extra protection.

Most headgear is adjustable. Make sure it fits snugly—you don't want it to "slide" and obstruct your vision as you spar. (A sure sign of a novice is loose headgear. It causes him to divert a great amount of energy to "sliding" his headgear back into its proper position.)

Good headgear, like boxing gloves, is "personal" equipment. It gets broken in over time until it comes to fit you perfectly, and it seems to last forever. So start out with a better model, which costs forty to forty-five dollars.

Mouthpiece. Never spar without a mouthpiece. In addition to protecting your dental work per se, a good mouthpiece prevents cuts inside the mouth and on the tongue.

Many pros get their mouthpiece custom-fitted by a dentist. If you are an owner of delicate bridgework, etc., you might consider a visit to your dentist as well. For most white-collar boxers, however, the "boil-and-mold"-type mouthpiece available at any sporting goods store works just fine. The price is right too, at about five dollars.

Wear your mouthpiece during your noncontact Boxer's Workout

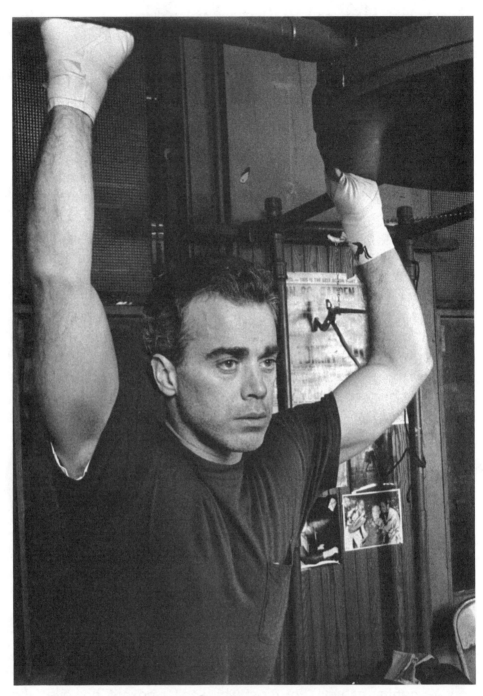

Joseph Carberry before a workout at the Gramercy. You can do the Boxer's Workout at a serious boxing gym, most fitness clubs, or in your own home gym or fitness area—pick the location that's right for you.

routine for several days before you spar. This way you'll get used to how it feels, and get comfortable breathing with it inside your mouth.

Keep your mouthpiece clean at all times. Many pros store their mouthpiece in a small plastic butter tub filled with mouthwash. As a result, the mouthpiece gradually loses its "rubber" taste and assumes that of the fighter's favorite mouthwash brand. Not as bothered by the "rubber" taste, the author simply stores his mouthpiece in a plastic sandwich bag and rinses it with water before insertion and after use.

Boxer's protective cup. In Little League, a protective cup meant a cheap plastic piece that snapped into your jock and covered your essentials and nothing more. A boxer's protective cup is more substantial: It is actually a leather "girdle." It provides protection from the navel on down, with the cup built in.

Boxer's protective cups start at about forty-five dollars—a minimal investment compared to the value of the family jewels.

HAND WRAPPING: PURPOSE AND METHOD

Purpose

Wrap your hands before every Boxer's Workout. As mentioned earlier, hand wraps protect your knuckles from abrasion and provide support for your wrist to combine your wrist and fist into one "unit." This reduces the chance of wrist injury and sprain, which can result if you bend your wrist as it strikes the heavy bag—or an opponent.

In addition to the physical protection, the wrapping of the hands has a ritualistic significance that you don't come across very often anymore. From Sullivan to Tyson to you, every fighter "gets wrapped" before he partakes of the sweet science. Out of respect for the legacy as well as the health of your knuckles, take a little time and practice until you get it right. Soon you'll be wrapping your hands as quickly and effectively as the pros.

Method

There are a variety of hand-wrapping techniques, each developed and championed by an individual trainer or group of trainers in view

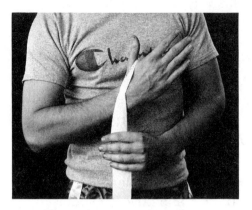

Place loop on thumb, as bandage falls across outside of wrist.

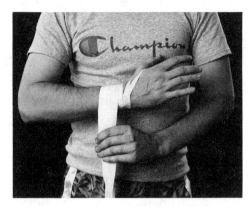

Wrap twice around wrist.

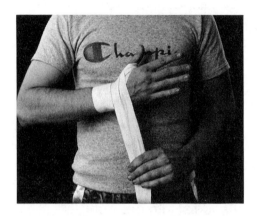

Wrap once around thumb.

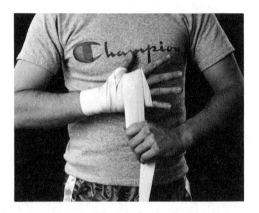

Wrap knuckles of flexed hand.

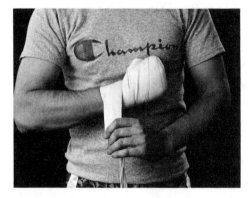

Finish wrapping wrist.

66

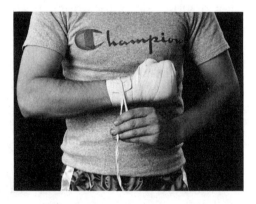

Tie tightly via bow knot.

of the previous considerations. The method photo-illustrated here comes from Al Gavin. In his more than twenty years of experience, Al has safely and effectively wrapped more hands, including the author's, than the number of hairs on anybody's head. His method is simple, straightforward, and perfect for the white-collar boxer.

Finally (as mentioned earlier) you might substitute elastic (Ace) bandages for the standard hand wraps shown here. It's the author's experience that they provide a "tighter wrap," without cutting circulation. Further, the end of an elastic bandage is secured more easily, because it can simply be tucked underneath the wrapped bandage itself; it doesn't need to be "tied off."

Overall, you want to wrap tight enough for support, but not so tight that you cut circulation. Within these parameters, follow the steps as shown at left.

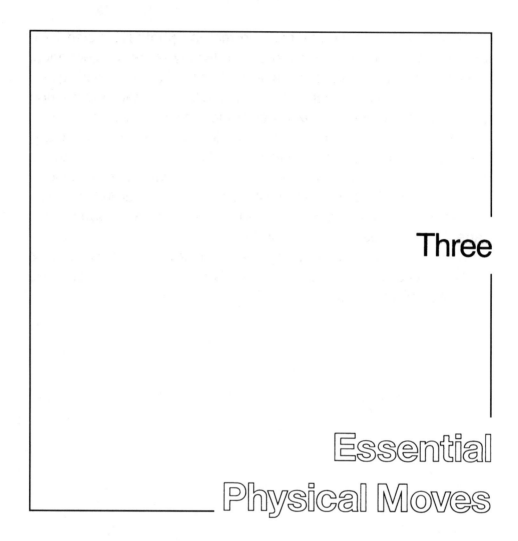

Three

Essential
Physical Moves

To gain maximum fitness, safety, and enjoyment from the Boxer's Workout, you should first have a basic understanding of boxing's essential moves and punches. This section presents them in a simple, straightforward manner. Use it as a ready reference guide during all phases of your program, from preconditioning right on through your regular execution of the Boxer's Workout (see Chapter Four), and prior to any sparring.

The photo illustrations include multiple-exposure photography where appropriate, to convey the entire range of motion for a given movement or punch in a way that single-exposure photographs usually can't. Single shots are also used, each isolating an important component of the larger movement.

It's important to know not only *what* to do, but *why* it is done that way. The photo illustrations for each move are, therefore, accompanied by a brief description of the purpose and thinking behind the move. The language gets a little graphic at points—for example, "The uppercut works best as an inside counterpunch delivered to the "hanging" head of a careless aggressor." However, it's essential that you fully understand the in-combat rationale for each move so that you can better execute it as you train—even if you never actually spar. (Similarly, martial artists and fencers practice combat-rooted "forms" against an imaginary opponent as an important part of training.)

Beyond that, the photos were painstakingly choreographed to do the majority of the "talking." Prop the book open so that you can view them easily as you practice. Whenever you're unsure about any aspect of a punch or move, check the photo.

A note to southpaws: Although the photo illustrations and text are biased toward right-handed boxers, the same principles and techniques apply to you, simply reversed. For example, you stand with your right foot forward, you generally move to your right, you jab with your right hand, and you throw a right hook.

KEYS TO BETTER PRACTICE

Relaxation is the single most important ingredient for the effective practice of the physical moves described in this chapter, and for the smooth, effective execution of the Boxer's Workout. Yet the majority of beginning boxers are anything but relaxed. Instead, they are overly concerned with how they look to others. This distracts their attention from the task at hand and "tightens them up," inhibiting performance and learning.

The author was no different: When I first began workouts at the Gramercy, I was simply "too tight" to improve quickly. I tensed my shoulders and flexed my arms unnecessarily, in an attempt to look more muscular and "macho." I carried myself in a chest-out, "top-heavy" manner which made me as rigid as a robot, caused me to rush and lunge, and wasted tremendous amounts of energy. (I could never understand why I was so exhausted after just a few rounds of work.) Ironically my "tightness," born out of an undue concern with looking good, actually made me look bad—a real "catch twenty-two."

Like anything else, you'll look and feel more relaxed with boxing's physical moves the more you practice them. In the meantime I offer the following interrelated body-and-mind training techniques. They helped me—and I believe they can help you—to stay relaxed, to execute better, and ultimately to progress more quickly.

Screen out spectators. This is especially true if you work out in a serious boxing gym. The majority of onlookers don't know good technique from bad. And the professionals you might be especially self-conscious in front of aren't looking at you anyway, by definition, they're completely focused on their own efforts. Concentrate fully on what you're doing, without diverting any energy to onlookers.

Find your "center" and move with it. Visualize your "center" at a spot about two inches below your navel, in between your belly and back. Be aware of your center from the moment you get into boxing stance. Move and punch with an awareness of your center. As better boxers and martial artists have known for years, "center awareness" helps keep you "grounded" yet flexible. It helps you to avoid top-heavy lunging, and keeps you relaxed and "on balance."

Concentrate on being relaxed. It sounds like a nonsequitur, but it isn't. If you feel yourself rushing or tightening up, simply pause, take a few deep breaths, and find your "center," and then slowly begin again. Don't punch too hard or too fast, especially during preconditioning. (Again, your muscles aren't ready yet.) Save full-speed, full-force punching for the heavy bag—and not until you've been doing the Boxer's Workout for at least several weeks.

For any given punch or movement, visualize the entire range of motion. Keep the multiple-exposure image in mind as you practice the individual components separately. Then execute the move through its full range of motion; first slowly, then faster—up to about medium speed. Visualizing the entire range of motion as you work on individual components will help you to move in a more fluid manner.

Practice without physically practicing. In keeping with the previous point, practice each move in your mind even when you're not

70

physically practicing. Toss this book in your briefcase and study this section on the train. Visualize yourself smoothly executing each of the moves, so that they gradually become second nature.

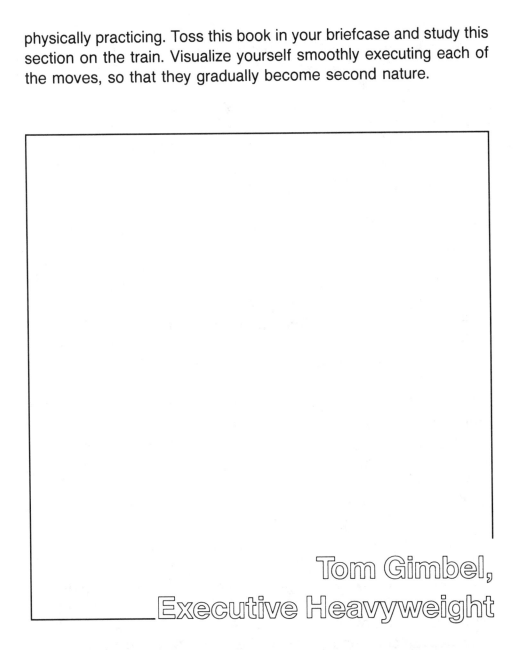

Tom Gimbel, Executive Heavyweight

Tom Gimbel is confidence. He walks into the gym with vibrancy and purpose (there's business to be taken care of here). He hits the heavy bag with a focused power that's downright intimidating, and this so impressed the author that I asked him to help choreograph and model the essential physical moves that appear on the following pages. Just as interesting as those boxing moves, however, is Tom Gimbel, the quintessential boxer/businessman.

Boxing runs in Tom's blood. It all started with his grandfather, Bernard F. Gimbel. Upon entering the University of Pennsylvania as an untried freshman, Bernard promptly dethroned the school's upperclassman heavyweight champion, and went on to represent U. of P. in intercollegiate boxing competition until his graduation. Bernard enjoyed a successful professional boxing career before going into business (Gimbel's department store). Highlights include service as a sparring partner for the great Philadelphia Jack O'Brien, who defeated none other than the great Bob Fitzimmons for the light-heavyweight championship of the world on December 20, 1905. Bernard was a close personal friend of Gene Tunney; the two sparred frequently. He remained on the boxing scene long after his competitive days, judging many important contests.

Tom's father David and his uncle Peter carried on the Gimbel fistic tradition, winning numerous amateur bouts as members of the Yale University boxing team. David went on to become a successful Wall Street financier—boxing remained an avocation until his tragic death, from cancer, at age twenty-nine. Peter's amateur career included a skirmish with Tommy (Hurricane) Jackson, the formidable heavyweight contender who lost a split decision to Floyd Patterson in the elimination tournament to determine a successor to Rocky Marciano. Peter later served as sparring partner for none other than George Plimpton as the latter, in the courageous spirit of participatory journalism, prepared for a three-round boxing exhibition with then light-heavyweight champion Archie Moore. Boxing remained Peter's sport of choice as he went on to become a noted film director and cinematographer (Blue Water, White Death and Andrea Doria: The Final Chapter).

And so it was with enthusiastic family support that young Tom first tasted the sweet science, taking time from his economics studies at Bowdoin College to whale away at the heavy bag. Solitary training sessions soon gave way to some sparring,

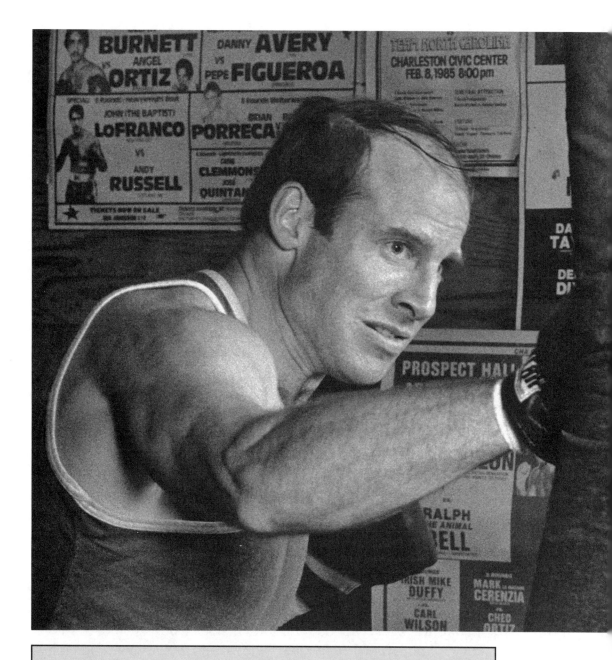

and his first boxing injury: "I broke my fourth metacarpal on top of someone's head." After a brief recovery period, during which he received his M.B.A. from Columbia University and began his finance career as an associate investment banker at a major-bracket firm, Tom resumed sparring. With a modicum of formal training to complement the formidable force generated by his

6'2", 215-pound frame, Tom entered the 1979 New York Golden Gloves competition.

Tom was encouraged at the time by a friend who was an ex-professional boxer. "He told me, 'Just hit these guys on the chin and you'll knock them out.'" That advice rang true during Tom's first match. "I knocked him out—really out." Tom also kayoed his next opponent, cutting him badly in the process. "I didn't know anything except to attack." In the quarterfinals Tom met a more experienced opponent who won the first two rounds by using an effective jab and defense: "He made me miss." Tom won the third and final round big, but lost the match on points. "I just couldn't put him away," he recalls apologetically.

Encouraged by his Golden Gloves experience, Tom began formal training under coach Vinny Ferguson, former NCAA and AAU national champion and an accomplished professional middleweight. (Vinny's father had trained Tom's dad and his uncle Peter.) Tom promptly won the New York Athletic Club heavyweight championship, which he was to hold for five years. It was sometime during this period that he was aptly dubbed "the Bomb," a nickname which was to stick throughout successful campaigns against the cream of the amateur crop in the New York metropolitan area.

Tom's amateur career peaked in 1983, when he fought his way to the prestigious Empire State Games as heavyweight champion of the Long Island region. At the games he surpassed a talented field of statewide representatives before losing in the championship match.

I asked Tom how at that point he faced the little voice that confronts every serious nonprofessional boxer—those with only a fraction of Tom's talent, those who would never admit it in a public place: "What if I put my career on hold for a year or two and took a shot at the professional game?" Tom answered with clinical precision, as if rendering judgment on a company's financial position, "I'd had quite a few amateur fights. I'd sparred in the gym with the best professionals, including a world champion and a North American champion. I knew I had what it takes to be a successful professional boxer—but not a world champion."

Tom remains active on the New York boxing scene, competing at the New York Athletic Club and in numerous charity events. (He won by knockout in the recent Wall Street Charity Fund bouts held at Madison Square Garden.) He trains and spars regularly: "I'm always within reach of boxing condition." He's married, with two children, and was recently named managing director at his firm.

It's not without some envy that the author notes that Tom Gimbel seems to have found the balance between family, career, and fitness which can be so elusive for the white-collar professional. Over several lunches in midtown Manhattan, he shared his unique perspective on the character and benefits of boxing. It became clear during our meetings that Tom's warmth and personal humor are accompanied by insights as crisply defined as his left hook. They appear below because they are important: a white-collar practitioner's view of a thinking man's sport as he experiences it. In Tom's words:

"The public at large looks at boxing as devoid of any art—two brutes slugging it out in a cage. Just the opposite, the sport is one of infinite subtlety, of physical and psychological refinement. The aspects of body choreography, balance, timing, and conditioning are on a par with those of a dancer or gymnast—or greater. The subtle feints, slips, footwork, weight transfer, the careful establishment of distance and range, and the almost undetectable (but intentional) bumps and pushes that result in superior position all contribute to the art of the sport.

"As essential as these refinements are, however, the importance of determination, durability, and power cannot be understated. Men like Rocky Marciano, Jack Dempsey, and Vito Antuofermo used these qualities to overcome more technically adept opponents. Other boxers, like Sugar Ray Robinson, Muhammad Ali, Roberto Duran, and Marvin Hagler, managed to put it all together as complete fighters during their prime years.

"The mental gamesmanship of the sport is as important as the physical aspects. It involves psychological operant conditioning, among other tactics. One boxer executes a given combination of punches several times, conditioning a certain defensive response. Then the boxer breaks his sequence by changing the last punch of the combination. The 'conditioned' opponent, who defended against a punch that never came, instead gets hit with the punch that replaced it in the combination.

"Finally, the better boxer knows himself—he uses his natural assets to his greatest advantage. The tall man with long reach wages war from long range. He circles his opponent continuously, using the expanse of the ring and a crisp jab to score hits and to confuse and tire his adversary. The shorter, more compact man seeks to fight at close quarters, where his long-limbed opponent can't punch as effectively. He uses the constraints of the ring to 'cut off' his opponent and 'bring the fight inside,' where he throws combinations of short punches.

"In no other sport can a single, perfectly timed and landed stroke win the entire contest, no matter how great the deficit. In few other sports is there such a blending of offense and defense, so that the avoidance maneuver becomes the first part of the attack. The high stakes of boxing offer a greater incentive for conditioning, since a missed parry results in a blow to the face. And in no sport is the difference between winning and losing so great: victory brings total elation, while losing is almost inconsolable.

"Boxing is an important part of my life. It keeps me in touch with physical reality. It's good for almost anyone, at any level of participation, from conditioning to competition. Boxing keeps you physically and mentally sharp, agile, quick, and conditioned —there's no room for sluggishness, slacking off, or anything but the utmost alertness.

"Boxing has a way of giving you confidence and humility at the same time. The confidence comes with knowing how to box, the humility from recognizing and being in the ring against better fighters. Rarely do you find a champion without some humble quality—he wasn't always king of the hill."

THE BALANCED STANCE

The balanced stance is the starting point for all boxing activity. If the stance is not executed correctly, it's very difficult to perform the essential physical moves of the sport: to mount an effective attack, to safely defend yourself. Spend some extra time and get your stance right—everything that follows will come much easier.

The stance presented here is the classic (orthodox) boxing stance, which has proven effective for the overwhelming majority of boxers from generation to generation. It is especially appropriate for the white-collar boxer because it is relatively easy to learn and offers the practitioner great safety. While it's true that unorthodox alternatives like Floyd Patterson's "peek-a-boo" and Joe Frazier's "crouch" were effective for those champions, unorthodox stances by definition remain the exception. They run counter to the physical attributes and/or capabilities of the majority of boxers, and are difficult to master unless patiently practiced under close supervision by a qualified trainer. It is recommended that you learn the classic stance described here before experimenting (under a trainer's supervision only) with any unorthodox alternatives.

Again, be aware of your "center" as you get into your stance and during subsequent movements and punches.

How to Stand

Place your feet comfortably apart. You should feel "on-balance"—sufficiently "set," yet able to move easily. Put your weight on the balls of your feet. This naturally raises your rear (right) heel, and to a lesser extent your front (left) heel. Put about the same amount of weight on each foot.

Bend your knees slightly. Not too much or you'll find yourself in a crouch, which can be awkward and tiring. Not too little either, or you'll limit the amount of power you can generate from your legs, as well as your shock absorption capability.

Position yourself sideways toward your opponent. With front foot, hip, and shoulder in line, you should be positioned sideways toward your opponent. This automatically puts your protective left

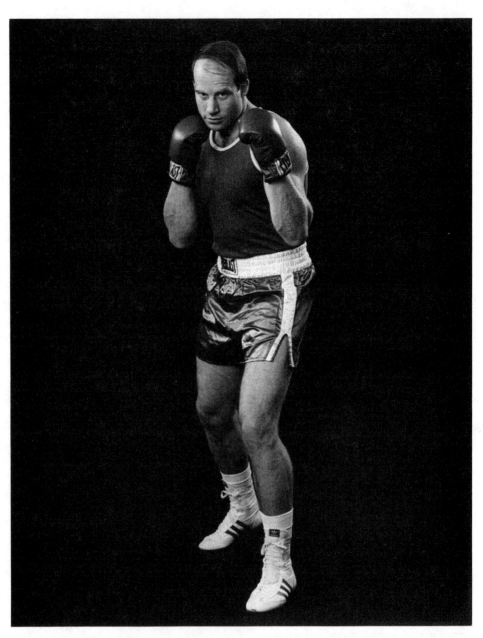

The balanced stance: front view.

hand between you and your opponent, maximizes your reach, and minimizes the amount of target area—that is, you—that is exposed.

Caution: Don't square your hips toward your opponent. This "opens up" your stance, giving your opponent a greater target area

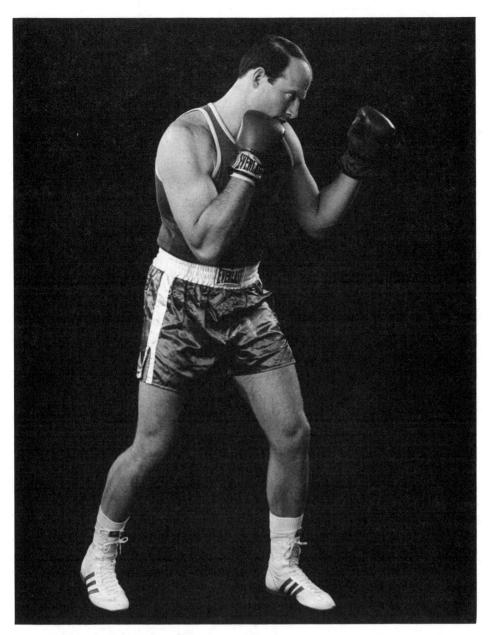

The balanced stance: side view.

and reducing your reach. Further, it necessarily results in your left hand being along your side, where it is less useful, instead of in front of you, where it can better protect your chin and body.

Position your right hand: fist close to chin, elbow close to

body. Note how the right fist is in position to protect the chin. The right elbow stays close to your ribs, perpendicular to the floor. From this position you'll realize maximum power when throwing your right and can easily protect your rib cage. Don't hold your right too high, or let your elbow flap out like a chicken wing, since this reduces your punching power and leaves your ribs dangerously exposed. Don't hold it too low either—it leaves your chin wide open for an opposing left hook.

Position your left hand: top of fist in line with top of shoulder, elbow slightly extended but still in position to protect your body. Note in the photos how the left fist is in ideal position to either jab or block. Similar to the right, the left elbow is roughly perpendicular to the floor. Keep your left up! Holding the left too low, as a result of fatigue, poor technique, or both, is the most common—and most dangerous—technical mistake made by novice boxers. Again, avoid the "chicken wing" tendency, as it reduces the power of your jab and leaves your midsection vulnerable to an opposing right.

Tuck your chin into your chest. This is slightly uncomfortable at first. But note in the side-view photo how the "tucked" chin is naturally protected by the left shoulder and right fist.

MOVEMENT

For boxers, knowing "how to move" in the ring is as important as knowing how to walk. Effective movement puts you in just the right position, at just the right distance, to effectively attack or defend. It conserves your energy. It helps you control the action.

As you attempt to perfect your movement, keep these factors in mind:

- Effective movement is relaxed. Easy and fluid. You should be no more self-conscious or "tight" than when you take a walk.
- Effective movement is controlled. No rushing or lunging. If you feel yourself losing control, simply pause, breathe, find your "center"; then begin again, more slowly.
- Effective movement is directed. It should reflect and help you achieve your strategic objective—that is, cut off the ring and force the action, score points by jabbing from a distance, etc.

80

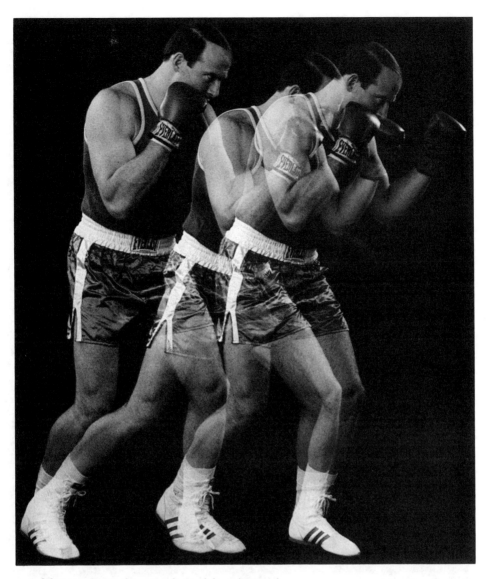

Movement: forward and backward.

• Effective movement is economical—no unnecessary bouncing, overstepping, or flash. These waste energy.

How to Move

Starting in the classic stance, the foot that should be moved first is the one in the direction you wish to go.

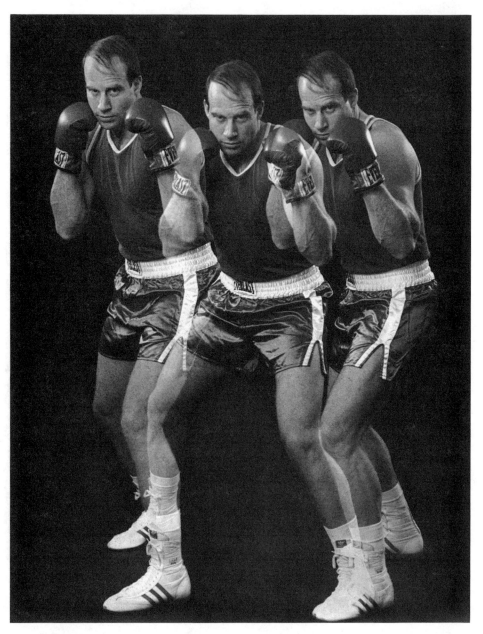

Movement: side to side.

• If you want to move forward, step first with your forward (left) foot; then follow with your back (right) foot. If you want to move backward, step first with your back (right) foot; then follow with your forward (left) foot.

82

· If you want to move left, step first with your left foot; then follow with your right foot. If you want to move right, step first with your right foot; then follow with your left.

The above method prevents you from crossing your feet, which is dangerous. Further, note that the energy (push) for each step necessarily comes from the ball of the opposite foot.

Stay on the balls of your feet. If you're up on your toes you're unstable; if you're flat-footed, you won't be able to move quickly enough.

Don't overstep. It puts you off balance.

Don't jump or bounce. At least one foot should be in contact with the floor at all times.

ADDITIONAL CONSIDERATIONS

Overall, maintain a distance from which you can "stick" your opponent with your jab; then either follow with your right or move away. You should generally move in the direction of your jabbing hand: If you're right-handed (that is, you jab with your left), you should generally move to your left. However, be sure to break the pattern periodically and move in the opposite direction—this prevents your opponent from "timing" you. More on the role of movement when we discuss the development of your personal boxing style.

THE LEFT JAB

Since your left hand is held closest to your opponent and the jab is thrown in a straight line, the left jab is your most direct means of contact with your adversary. As a result, it is the most important and most frequently used punch in your repertoire.

The jab works like an antenna, helping you to "feel" where your opponent is, to precisely measure his distance. When you're on the attack, it is the first punch in the majority of combinations available to you. It drives your opponent backward and off balance, and partially obscures his vision—setting him up for additional, more telling blows. When you're on defense, your jab keeps your opponent at a

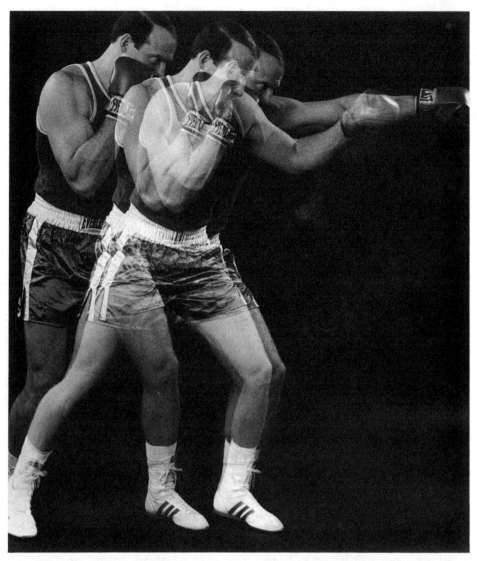

The left jab: multiple exposure, open-side view through full extension.

safe distance and hinders his ability to "set up" and throw punches effectively.

Although the number of jabs you throw depends on your individual style, you can expect that a minimum of sixty percent of your punches will be left jabs. (Even boxers with an "infighting" style rely heavily on an effective jab.) The jab thus deserves a major emphasis as you practice your punching technique.

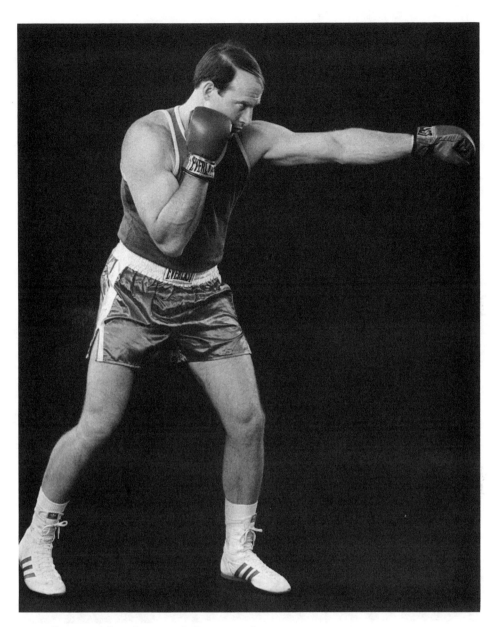

Open-side view at full extension.

How to Throw the Left Jab

Drive off the ball of your back (right) foot as you step forward. Although the jab is a "snapping" punch, the body's full force

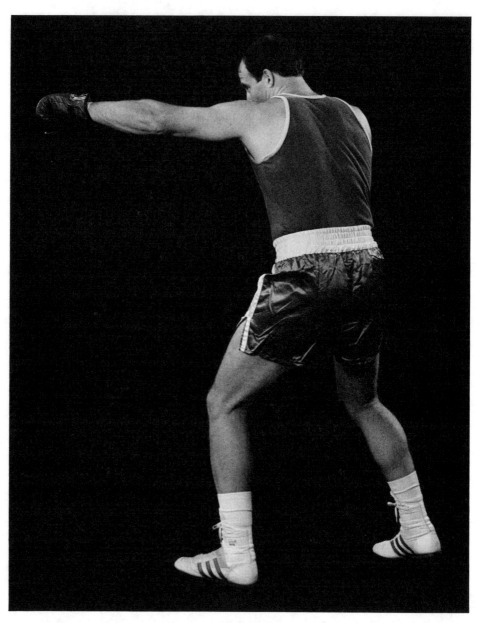

Closed-side view at full extension.

should be behind it. This is achieved largely as a result of "driving off" the ball of your back (right) foot.

Rotate your left shoulder and fist as you execute the punch. Your shoulder should rotate and your fist should "turn over" as the jab is delivered. The shoulder rotation significantly extends your

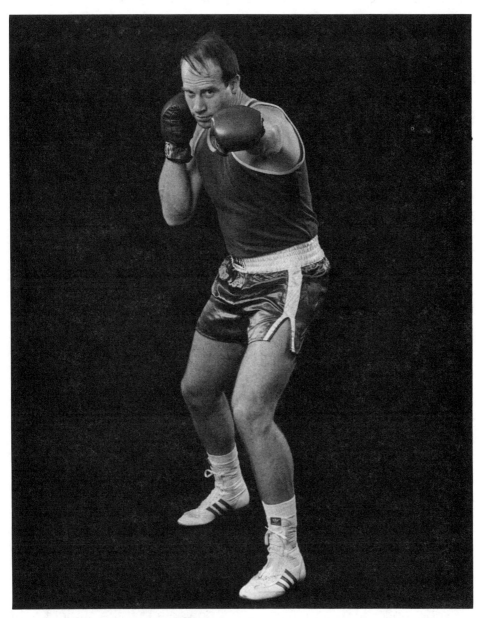

Straight-on view at full extension.

reach and provides greater protection for your "tucked" chin. The rotation of your fist increases your force on impact.

Punch in a straight line. Don't "loop" or "curve" your delivery. The jab is a "straight" punch.

Make sure your arm is fully extended at impact. Your elbow should be "locked" to maximize power and give the punch its "snapping" character.

Punch "through" your opponent. Visualize and deliver the jab "through" your opponent rather than terminating your force at the point of impact—that is, "pulling" your punch.

Keep your right hand in correct position as you jab with your left. "Dropping the right" is a common beginner's mistake that leaves you vulnerable to a left-hand counterpunch. Check your form.

After follow-through, quickly return your left hand to its proper position. Be careful not to let your left arm dangle. (Boxers call this "letting the left 'lay.'") Promptly return your left hand to classic-stance position along the same straight-line path on which the jab was delivered. This protects you against opposing counterpunches and puts you back on balance so you can follow with additional punches of your own, or move away.

ADDITIONAL CONSIDERATIONS

Use your jab as the "feeler" it is intended to be. When you want to "move in," do so behind your jab. When you want to "buy time," jab and circle away. Vary the speed and frequency of your jab. This keeps your opponent off guard and prevents him from "timing" you. Double up on your jab now and then by launching a second jab just before your left hand is fully back in position. Bend your knees a bit more and jab at your opponent's body occasionally. If he lowers his hands, follow with a jab to his chin.

THE STRAIGHT RIGHT

If you're right-handed, the straight right is your "power" punch. The conventional explanation for this power is that the straight right "has your body behind it." That's true, but only as far as it goes— the fact is that *every* punch should have your body behind it, with the force originating from the ball of the proper foot and terminating "through" your opponent. The more precise reason for the power of the straight right is that the punch is delivered with the full and simultaneous rotation of your hips and shoulders, with the left side of your body working like a hinge.

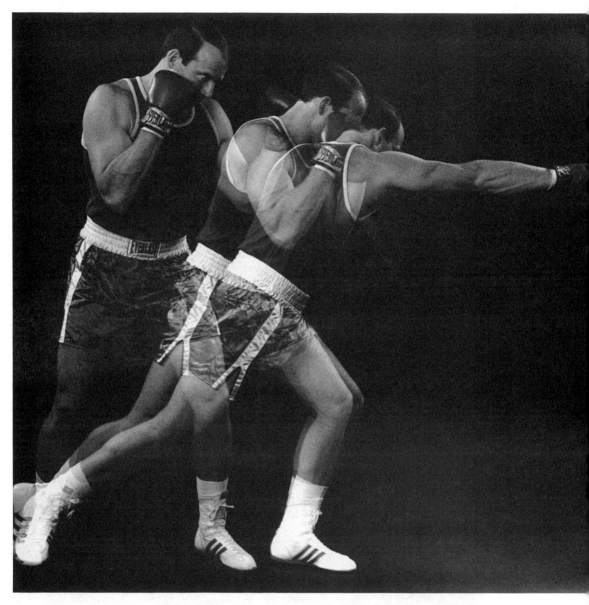

The right cross: multiple exposure, closed-side view through full extension.

The greater power of the straight right is not without a commensurately greater risk. If you miss, you are easily victimized by left-hand counterpunches as you struggle to regain your balance. What's more, you'll have spent a great deal of energy without a payoff. So before you throw a straight right, be reasonably sure that

89

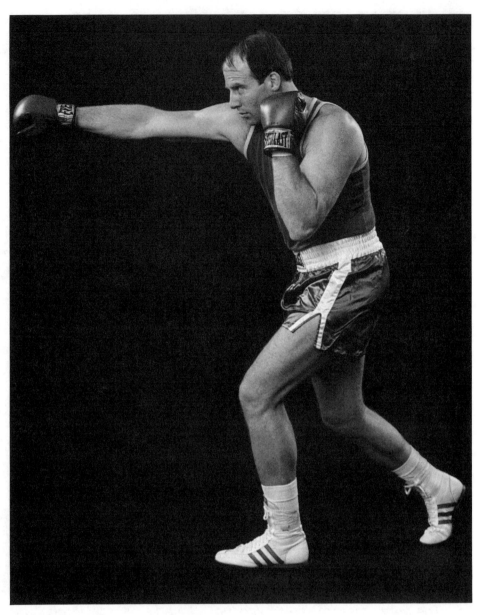

Open-side view at full extension.

it's going to land. "Set it up" by first throwing a left jab or double jab or by so accurately "timing" your opponent's pattern of movement that he can't help but "walk into" your straight right lead.

Finally, the terms "straight right" and "right cross" are used interchangeably by the man in the street and by a surprising number of

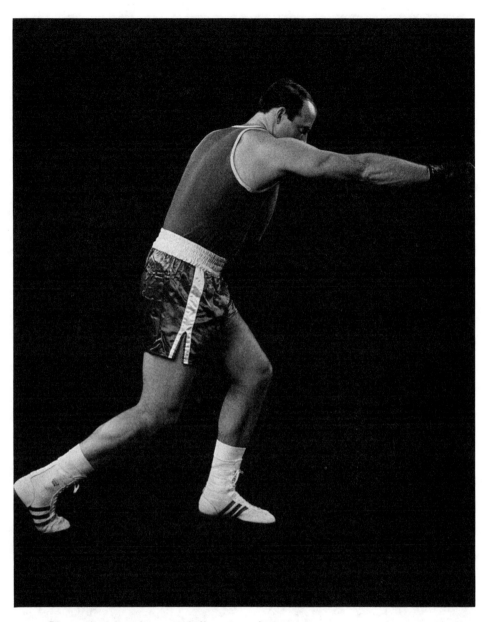

Closed-side view at full extension.

boxing people. However, they are not the same. While the straight right by definition follows a straight-line path to its target, the right cross is a counterpunch which is thrown with a slight arc over and across your opponent's left jab. The right cross is more difficult to execute because you must launch it while simultaneously "slipping"

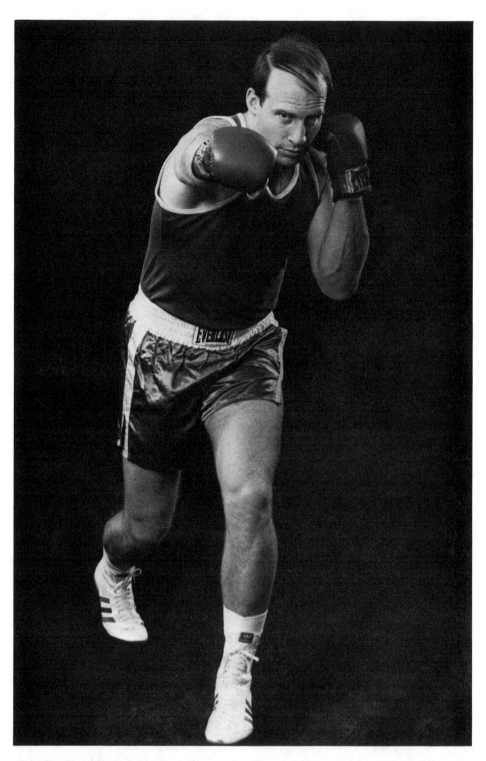

Straight-on view at full extension.

the opposing left jab. (If you don't time your "slip" perfectly, you'll wind up "eating" a left jab as your right cross goes awry.) It is recommended that at this beginning stage you concentrate primarily on developing an effective straight right.

How to Throw the Straight Right

Drive off the ball of your right foot while stepping forward with your left foot. The step forward can take place either on its own, as shown, or as part of a preceding left jab. (In the latter case the straight right would be the second punch in the classic one-two combination.)

With the left side of your body working like a hinge, simultaneously rotate your right hip and shoulder toward your opponent as you fully extend your right arm. At full-extension your right shoulder should be closer to your opponent than your left shoulder, and your hips should be fully squared.

Similar to the jab:

- Your fist "turns over" during delivery.
- Your arm is fully extended and your elbow is "locked" at impact.
- The punch is delivered in a straight line (as mentioned above).
- The punch is delivered "through" your opponent.

Be sure your chin is "tucked" throughout execution, for maximum protection. Your head moves from right to left, with the punch.

Don't lower your left arm as you throw your right. This would leave you vulnerable to a right-hand counterpunch.

Don't "telegraph" your right by pulling your arm back and "winding up" before you throw it.

After follow-through, **quickly return your right hand to its proper position** as you pivot back into classic stance.

ADDITIONAL CONSIDERATIONS

Don't get "right-hand-happy." Novices invariably throw too many straight right leads, which are easily defended. Instead, work to deliver the straight right as the more powerful portion of a one-two combination, after a left jab has first driven your opponent backward and partially blocked his vision.

THE LEFT HOOK

It was in one lightning instant on the evening of March 8, 1971, that Joe Frazier reached the zenith of his brilliant career, landing his "smoking" left hook on the jaw of the Greatest, whose protective right hand was well out of position at the moment of impact. Muhammad Ali struggled to his feet and after the mandatory eight-count miraculously pressed on.

There is no punch in boxing with as much romance as the left hook. And there is no punch as misunderstood. Many would-be "Smokin' Joes" hook wildly, or without power, or from too far away. These errors are due to a lack of knowledge of the mechanics of the punch and when to use it. As described below, the hook's power comes through the hooking arm rather than from it. And the punch is best delivered from in close, over your opponent's low right hand. From this range it can be launched by itself (as illustrated), used as a "finisher" after your straight right has driven your opponent backward, or used as an effective counterpunch after you've slipped outside an opposing straight right.

While the left jab can be delivered more quickly, and the straight right usually brings home more force, the left hook offers the element of surprise: if executed correctly, it usually travels outside your opponent's field of vision—he rarely gets a chance to make a meaningful countermove before impact. This makes the left hook particularly devastating, an "equalizer" which can instantly change the course of events.

How to Throw the Left Hook

- Working from the classic stance, dip your right knee slightly and square your hips toward your opponent.
- Transfer your weight to the ball of your left (front) foot as you begin your pivot and launch the punch.
- Rotate your hips and shoulders from square to sideways toward your opponent as you continue to pivot through delivery. This rotation during pivot creates significant power.

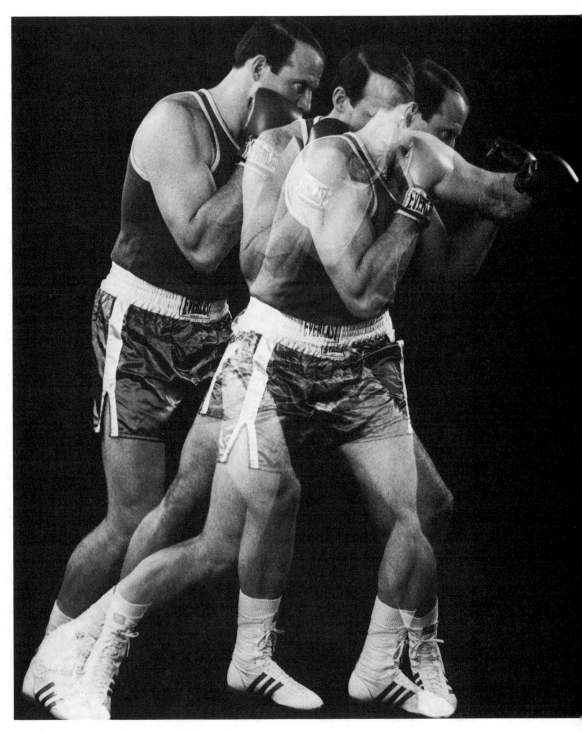

*The left hook: multiple exposure, open-side view through full
extension.*

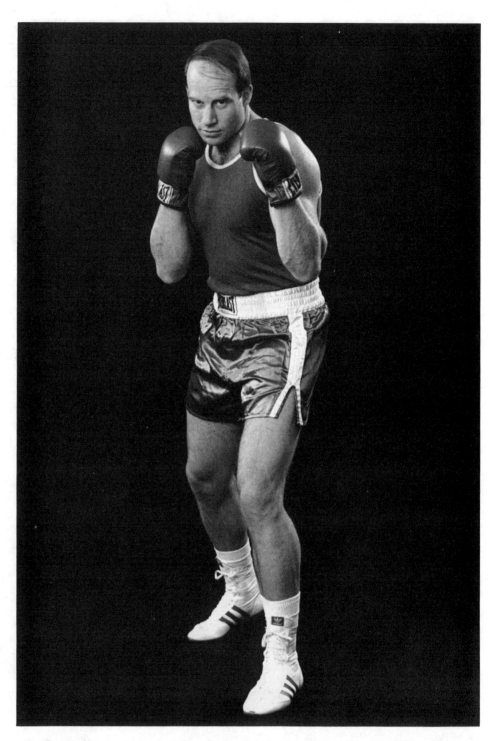

Straight-on view of the balanced stance, prior to the onset of the left hook.

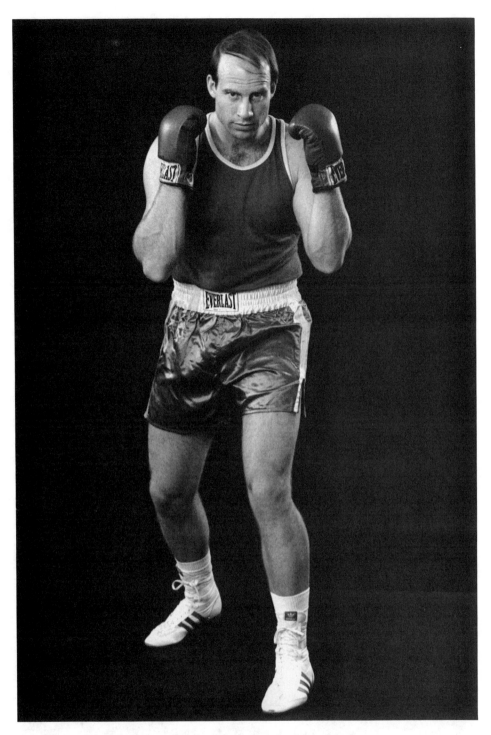

The onset of the left hook: straight-on view.

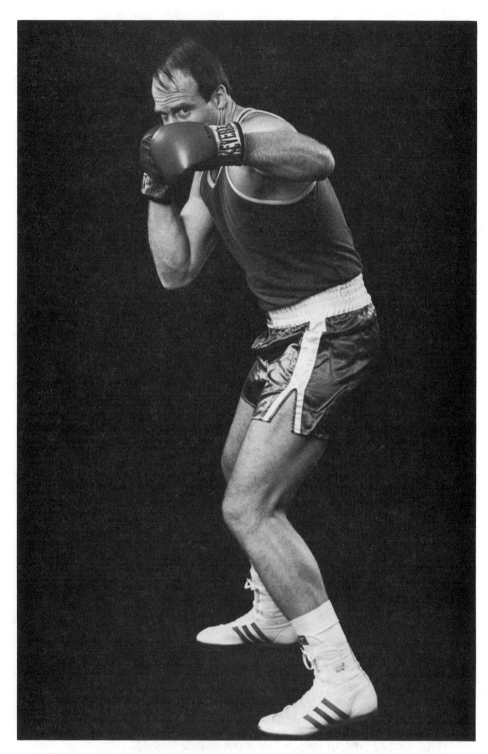

The hook at mid-extension: straight-on view.

98

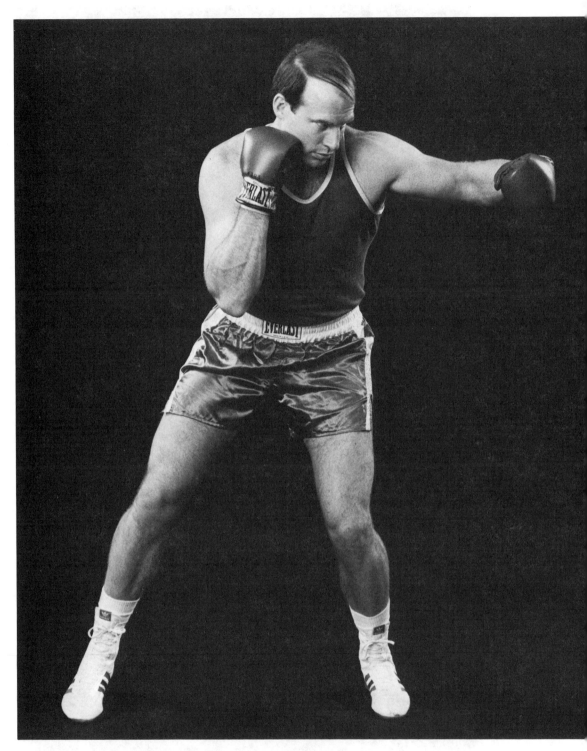

The hook at mid-extension: open-side view.

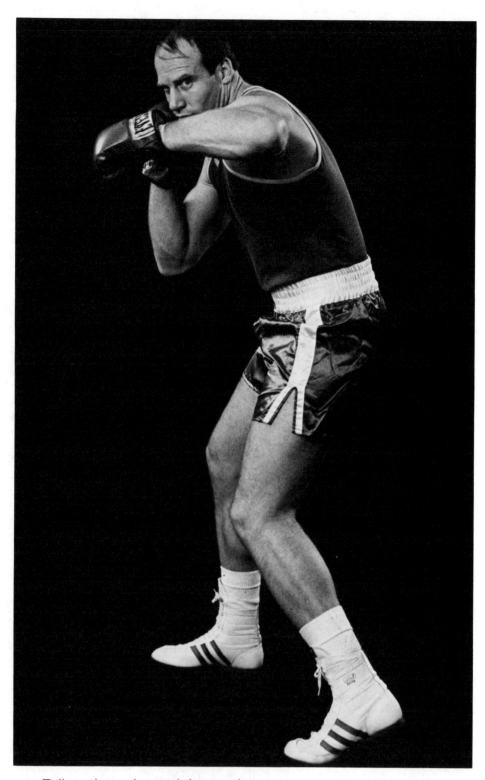

Follow-through: straight-on view.

100

- Keep the inside of your left (hooking) elbow parallel to the floor, with the elbow bent at a ninety-degree angle, as shown.
- As you follow through, keep your head down. Your "tucked" chin is protected by your right fist and left shoulder.
- Your head moves from left to right, with the punch.
- Again, be sure to deliver the blow "through" your opponent.

ADDITIONAL CONSIDERATIONS

Similar to the straight right, don't throw this punch indiscriminately. Work to set it up. Even though the hook is best thrown at close range, make sure you're not too close—this will result in your "wrapping" the punch around the back of your opponent's neck.

Try to develop a hook off the jab: step in with your left hook after you've driven your opponent back with your jab. Speed is the key here—very few boxers are fast enough to jab and then hook without getting tagged with a right-hand counter before their hook reaches its destination. Practice on the heavy bag until you're convinced you can execute it quickly enough to give it a try in sparring.

Finally, if you're right-handed, don't even *think* about hooking with your right. Your right hand is too far away from your target and completely visible during delivery. You'll more than likely "eat" a straight left counter before your right hook "nonpunch" is even halfway to its destination. Forget about the right hook—instead, work on developing your straight right and left hook.

THE UPPERCUT

The uppercut completes your portfolio of punches. Like the left hook, this punch is best delivered from close range. Unlike the hook, however, the uppercut can be thrown effectively with either hand.

The uppercut works best as an inside counterpunch delivered to the "hanging" head of a careless aggressor. Better boxers develop their uppercut counter to a point where it's practically instinctive: At the moment their opponent's head "hangs down," their uppercut "goes up." The uppercut can also serve as a telling body blow when driven "through" your opponent's solar plexus during infighting.

101

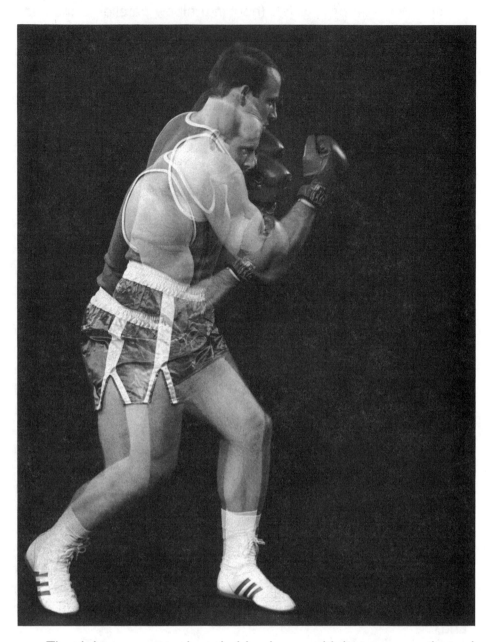

The right uppercut: closed-side view, multiple exposure through full extension.

How to Throw the Right Uppercut

- Working from the classic stance, bend your right knee and lower your right shoulder as you assume a crouching position.

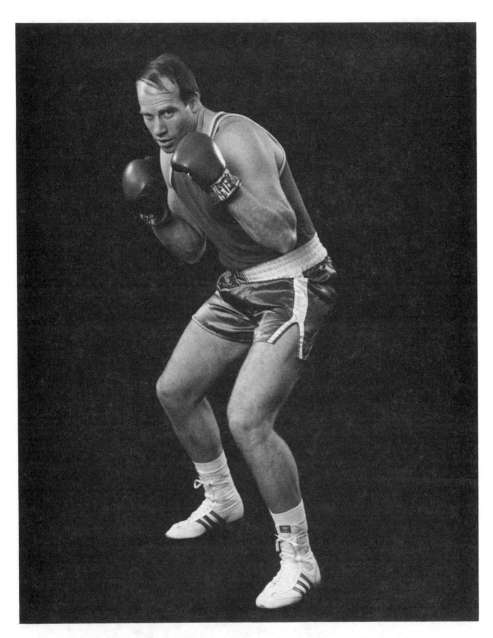

The onset of the right uppercut: straight-on view.

- Drive off the ball of your right foot as you rotate your hips toward your opponent.
- For maximum power, your elbow should be bent at a right angle during delivery and follow-through.
- Keep your left hand in protective position throughout execution.

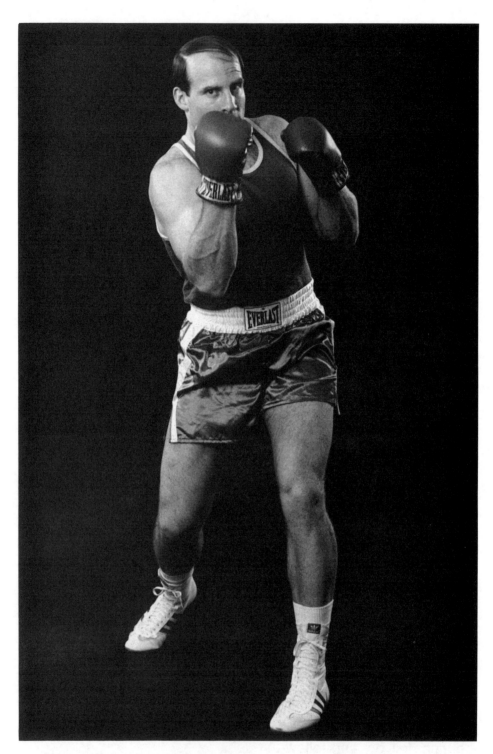

Right uppercut at full extension: straight-on view.

- Working from the classic stance, square your hips, bend your left knee, and lower your left shoulder as you transfer your weight to the ball of your left foot.
- Drive off the ball of your left foot as you deliver the punch, and rotate your hips back to their original sideways-to-opponent position. Note that this sideways-to-opponent finishing position contrasts with that of the right uppercut, which leaves your hips square to your opponent. These different finishing positions call for different follow-up punches, as described below.

ADDITIONAL CONSIDERATIONS

Uppercuts to the head tend to "stand up" your opponent. Follow a right uppercut to the head with a left hook to the head. This completes your combination and puts you back on balance. Follow a left uppercut to the head with a straight right to the head.

Uppercuts to the body tend to cause your opponent to lean forward—step back and follow with an uppercut to his "hanging" head.

Don't throw uppercuts from far outside: (1) they take forever to reach their destination and are thus easily "picked up" by your opponent; (2) they leave you wide open for an opposing straight punch, which can reach your chin well before your outside uppercut reaches your opponent's; and (3) even if your outside uppercut does land, it will have significantly less power than one thrown from inside; since your elbow will not be bent at the ninety-degree angle necessary to fully transfer the force from your body.

COMBINATIONS

The better boxer is not one-dimensional. He thinks in terms of landing multiple punches to multiple locations in logical and varying sequence. While you might have a left hook that you swear can send any mortal man to the moon, don't become a "one-punch fighter." Instead, work to perfect each of the punches previously demonstrated. And make your inevitable "favorite" punch even more effective by delivering it within a combination, where your preceding punches can camouflage it and ensure that your opponent is off balance when it is delivered.

How to Throw Effective Combinations

Order your punches in a way that keeps you on balance. One punch should naturally set up the next—the same way one shot sets up the next in a game of pool—with successive punches putting you back on balance. For example, you'll notice that as you complete the straight right, you're in good position to launch the left hook, which in turn puts you back on balance and leaves you in a "closed" or protected position from which you can fire additional punches or easily move away.

"Double up" on a jab or hook occasionally. Just about when you think your opponent figures that you never throw the same punch twice in a row (because you've observed the previous point), "double up" on a jab or hook. However, you should recognize that "doubling up" takes extra time, since you need to return to near-starting position to launch the (same) punch again. Practice doubling up on the heavy bag before you try it during sparring.

Think "head-body" to create and exploit openings. If you direct your attack at your opponent's head, you'll notice that he will tend to hold his hands higher. This leaves his body open. Similarly, if you work his body, he'll eventually lower his hands, exposing his head. Exploit these tendencies by taking a "head-body approach" as you throw combinations. A case in point is Joe Frazier, who worked his opponent's body consistently in order to wear him down and get him to lower his hands. Then, at precisely the right moment, Frazier would launch a left hook to the head.

Work feints into your combinations. By causing your opponent to react to a punch you don't throw, you can create an opening for the one you do. Feint by starting the "bait" punch only enough to draw the desired reaction. Then launch the punch you actually intend to throw. In general, set up right-handed punches by feinting with your left, and vice-versa; and set up body punches by feigning head punches, and vice-versa. Examples: Feign a left jab to the chin and step in with a straight right to the midsection, followed by a left hook to the head. Feign a straight right to the head and step in with a left hook to the body, followed by a left hook to the head.

Vary the pattern and speed of your punches, to avoid being "timed" by your opponent. Don't be predictable. Even slight variations will keep your opponent honest. For example: Throw successive left jabs at only three-quarters speed. Just when your opponent has gotten lulled into believing that your (intentionally) slow jab is the best you've got to offer, step in with the real thing and follow with a straight right and a left hook.

Factor your best punch into your thinking. There are two ways to do this: You can plan your combinations to "set up" your best punch and deliver it as the "finisher" in your sequence. Conversely, you can feign your best punch in order to land other blows more effectively. For example, if you've developed a reputation around the gym as a "pretty good left-hooker," during your next sparring session try feigning the hook and instead throwing your straight right.

Consider your opponent's characteristics and style. Without overreacting, ask yourself whether your opponent's physical characteristics and/or boxing style suggest certain combinations or series of combinations. Is he a stocky boxer who tends to bore in? Step back and throw an uppercut to his chin, followed by a left hook to his head. Is he a tall man who relies primarily on his jab? Step in with combinations to his body and "chop him down." Is he primarily a counterpuncher? Feint in order to draw his counterpunch; then counter his counter.

Get back on balance quickly. As stated previously, you should order the punches in your combination so that you finish on balance. Unless you're Superman, however, there will be times when you'll find yourself overcommitted and off balance. This is especially true when you miss a straight right. Don't panic. Don't stay in the overcommitted position as if you're posing either. Quickly pivot back into classic stance, take a deep breath, and find your center; then begin again.

Many boxers have enjoyed great success by executing these classic combinations supremely well.

Left jab–straight right (see photos below and at right). This is the classic one-two. The left jab drives your opponent backward and partially obscures his vision. The straight right delivers great power.

The left jab–straight right–left hook combination.

The left jab drives the opponent backward and partially obscures his field of vision.

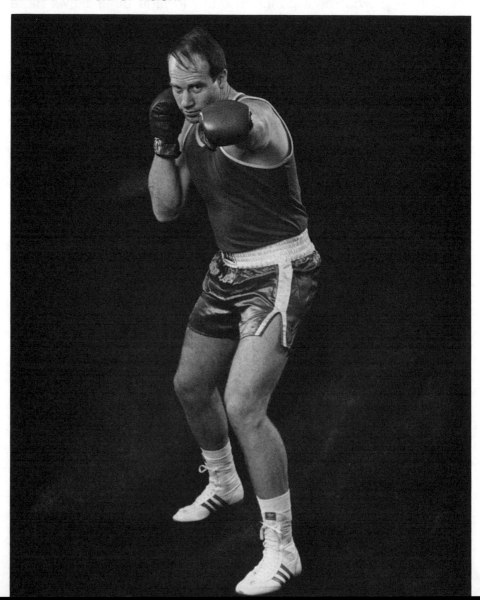

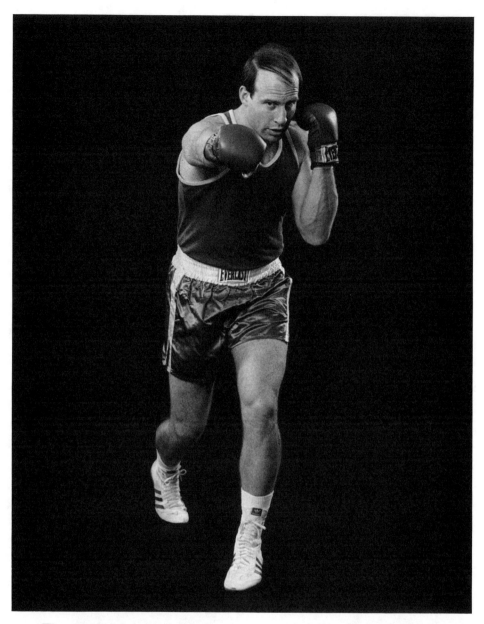

The straight right delivers great power and completes the "one-two" portion of the combination.

Left jab–straight right–left hook (see photos left, above, next page). This combination calls for you to follow the one-two with a left hook, delivered to either the body or chin. The hook puts you back on balance. From here you can easily move away or throw

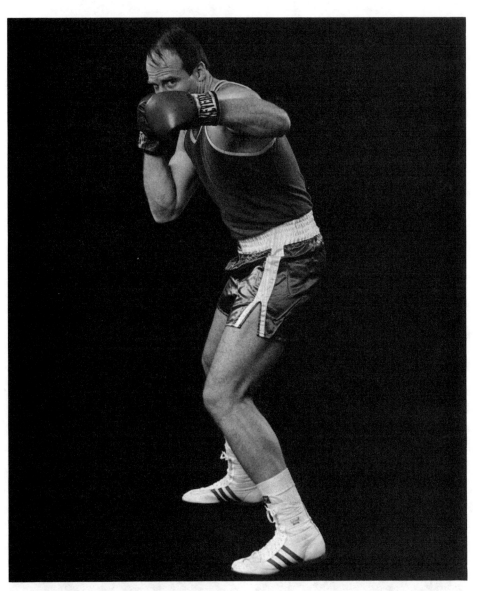

The left hook puts you back on balance.

additional punches—specifically a right uppercut to the body followed by another left hook to the head. Occasionally, feign the left jab and make the straight right your first punch in the combination.

Right uppercut–left hook. Again, the right uppercut works well when delivered to the head of a careless infighter. It tends to "stand up" your opponent, leaving him vulnerable to a left hook to the head.

Left jab–left hook–straight right–left hook. "Hooking off the jab" is effective yet difficult to master. Speed is of the essence.

Left jab–left hook to body–left hook to head–straight right. Practice "double hooking" on the heavy bag until you can do it quickly and powerfully; then finish with a straight right.

Left jab–right uppercut to solar plexus–left hook to chin. Step forward with the uppercut after you've driven your opponent backward with the jab. This combination reflects the "head and body" approach discussed earlier.

Left uppercut to solar plexus–straight right to head. This combination should be delivered from close range.

ADDITIONAL CONSIDERATIONS

Practice the combinations presented here until they become second nature: you'll want them to simply "flow" when you spar. Visualize your opponent as you practice. "See" him reacting to your punches. Observe and act on openings for subsequent punches. Be creative: improvise additional combinations on the heavy bag, with successive blows putting you back on balance. Finally, be patient: effective combination punching takes lots of practice.

Additional combinations will be presented when we discuss counterpunching, in the following section.

OPPORTUNISTIC DEFENSE

You've got to master the art of defense, or the most you can hope to be is a fighter—not a boxer. Some boxers (for example, Wilfred Benitez, the late Salvador Sanchez, and Jimmy Young) enjoyed tremendous success due primarily to their defensive skills. With rare exceptions their opponents found themselves missing punches, overcommitted, out of position—and ultimately victimized by a series of perfectly placed counterblows. Even boxers known for an attacking style (for example, Roberto Duran) rely heavily on effective defensive moves and counterpunches.

Superior defense is opportunistic. It sets up a counterpunch or series of counterpunches which can immediately turn the tables and put the attacker on the defensive. In ascending order of difficulty,

111

the three basic defensive moves are blocking, parrying, and slipping. You should strive to perform each of these smoothly. And you should learn how to capitalize on the opportunities they create by throwing appropriate counterpunches and counterpunch combinations. Since your defensive moves and counterpunches are every bit as important as your offensive moves, you should practice them just as much.

General Guidelines

Maintain your classic stance. As previously discussed, it inherently provides a great deal of protection: your hands are positioned to protect your head, pick off punches, and counterpunch. Your forearms and elbows are positioned to protect your body, and your chin is safely "tucked." Again, keep your hands up! This is the single most important component of effective defense.

Move and jab. Moving forward and backward alone isn't enough —you'll be easily "timed" and hit. Move from side to side as well. Flick your jab frequently. This will keep your opponent off balance and at a safe distance, so that he can't "set up" and throw effective punches.

Vary your defensive moves and counters. For any given punch your opponent might throw at you, there are generally several ways to effectively defend and counter. Try not to use the same move and counterpunch every time—if your opponent is smart, he'll feint to draw your (predictable) reaction, then nail you after you've committed.

Don't hesitate with your counterpunches. After you make your defensive move (block, parry, or slip), you'll have no more than a fraction of a second to counterpunch. If you hesitate, your opponent will simply hit you with the next punch in his combination.

Counterpunch in combination. This will enable you to take full advantage of your off-balance opponent.

The Three Basic Defensive Moves

Blocking. Blocking a punch is the easiest of the three basic defensive moves because it is the most instinctive. If you knew noth-

112

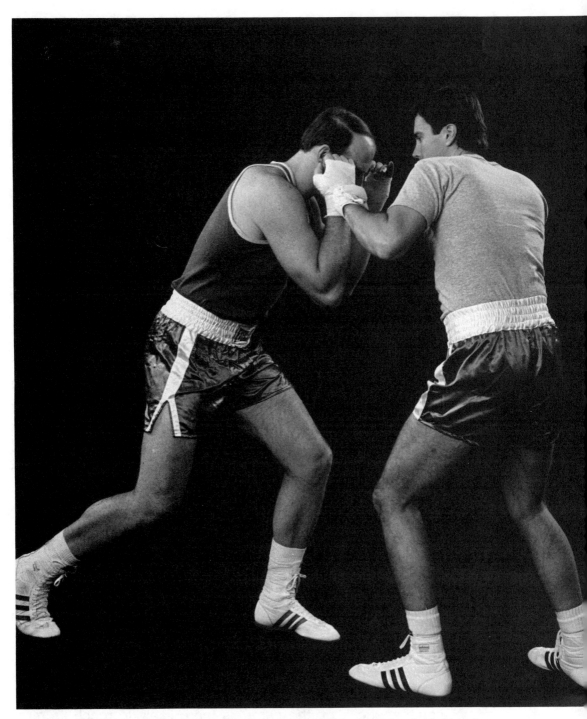

Blocking: Tom Gimbel blocks a left hook with his right hand. Tom's "opponent" is Brant Thomas, financial analyst, Office of Management and Budget, City of New York.

113

ing at all about boxing and someone threw a punch at your nose, you'd quickly raise a hand to block it, without even thinking about it. Blocking is considered the "safest" defensive move for the novice, simply because it is the one he is most likely to execute successfully.

The lower risk of blocking is of course accompanied by a commensurately lower "reward." Compared to parrying and slipping (the two remaining defensive moves), there's literally "less you can do" to your opponent after you've completed a block. For the novice, the blocking hand is basically "used up" and unavailable for counterpunching. Although you'll eventually learn to "punch off the block," you'll need lots of practice before you can do so with quickness and accuracy. Further, after blocking a straight punch you're necessarily farther away from your opponent than if you had parried or slipped the blow—you'll need to step forward in order to get close enough to counter effectively.

HOW TO BLOCK

In keeping with the classic stance, use your fist or the outside part of your wrist to block a punch to your head, and your forearm or elbow to block a punch to your body. Use only one hand to block any given punch. Blocking with both hands is unnecessary, and hinders your ability to counterpunch. The photo on page 113 shows Tom Gimbel blocking an oncoming left hook.

Parrying. To fend off straight punches, parrying is generally better than blocking: the parry actually redirects the oncoming blow, while the block can at best only neutralize it. Like the block, the parry "occupies" one hand. However, its "redirection" characteristic gives the parry four important advantages over the block:

- It provides a more open line of fire for your counterpunches, since your opponent's hand is moved "out of your way."
- It puts you in a better position to throw inside counterpunches. Since your forward movement need not stop at the end of the oncoming punch, it's easier to step inside as you parry.
- A counterpunch "off the parry" is more likely to reach its mark than one "off the block," since the parry brings your (parrying) hand slightly closer to your opponent.

114

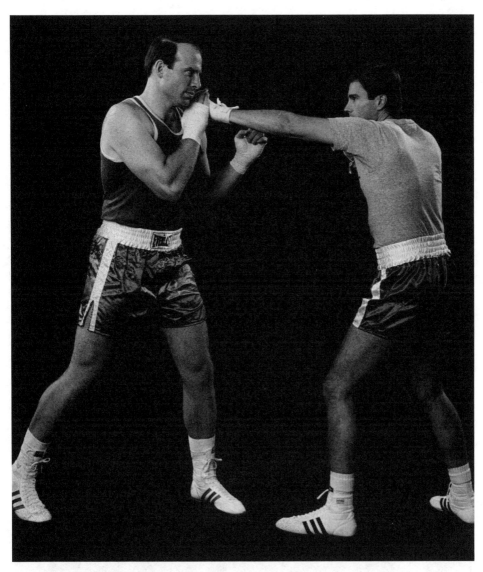

Parrying: using the right hand to parry a left jab.

- A parry is more likely to put your opponent off balance, since it reroutes his force in a direction he didn't intend it to go.

HOW TO PARRY

Parry an oncoming blow by simply "catching" it and pushing it aside and downward, out of your way. The photo above shows Tom Gimbel parrying a left jab; the photo on page 116 shows him parrying a right uppercut.

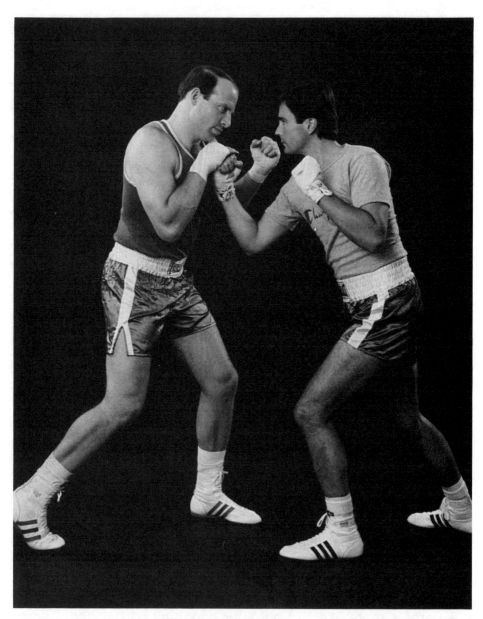

Parrying: using the right hand to parry a right uppercut.

Slipping. The better the boxer, the more he "slips" opposing punches. While slipping is the riskiest of the defensive moves and the most difficult to master, it is also the most effective:

• It leaves both your hands completely free to counterpunch, so

116

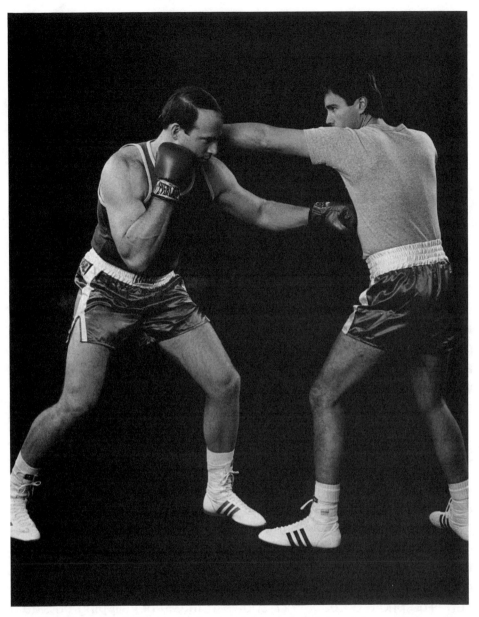

Slipping: Tom Gimbel slips outside a left jab and counters with a left to the body.

there are more counterpunches available to you, and it's easier to counterpunch in combination.

- Your counterpunches cannot be obstructed by your opponent's punching hand. His (extended) arm is well out of your line of fire.

117

- It puts you at an ideal distance from which to launch inside counterpunches. Since the opposing punch "goes by" you, it's much easier to step inside.
- It enables you to get off your counterpunches more quickly. The slip best enables you to fuse your defense and counterpunch into one efficient move, with your (defensive) slip serving as the first (launching) part of your counterpunch. This contrasts with counterpunching off the block or off the parry, both of which are more "two-step" in nature.
- Of the three defensive moves, it is the most frustrating to your opponent. Not only have you negated his punch, you're not even there anymore. What's more, you're in a perfect position to turn the tables with effective counterpunches—suddenly he's on the defensive.

Compared to blocking or parrying, the slip calls for quicker reaction: to be effective you'll need to start the slip sooner, before the punch has fully reached you. At the same time, it's important not to anticipate a punch and begin your slip too soon—a savvy opponent will feint to draw your slip, then hit you with a (different) blow as you slip the one he never threw.

HOW TO SLIP

Slip a punch by bending at the waist and knees (as shown on pages 117 and 119), so that you just avoid the oncoming blow and are in a perfect position to counterpunch. You can slip inside or outside an oncoming punch. Using an opposing left jab to your chin as an example, slip inside the punch by moving to your left such that the punch travels over your right shoulder. Slip outside the punch by moving to your right so that the punch travels over your left shoulder. (The photo on page 117 shows Tom Gimbel slipping outside a left jab. The photo at right shows him slipping inside a straight right.)

Slipping inside the punch usually leaves you in a better position to counterpunch, but it is at the same time the more difficult move. Further, an inside slip necessitates that you counterpunch especially quickly—or you'll get tagged with your opponent's opposite hand. Note photo, page 119: now that Tom's slipped inside the right, he must quickly fire a straight right of his own, or he'll get hit

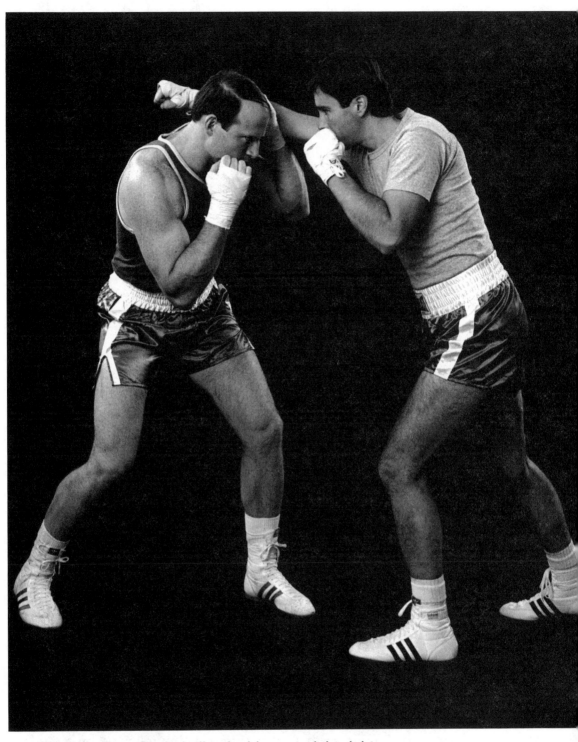

Slipping: Tom Gimbel slips inside a straight right.

with an opposing left. For this reason it's best to fuse your slip and counterpunch into one move, as described previously.

Keep your hands up (in classic stance position) as you slip. This leaves you better protected in case you mistime the move, and it enables you to counterpunch more effectively.

Slip only enough to avoid the blow. Don't "overslip"—it leaves you out of position and off balance, and wastes energy.

DEFENSIVE MOVE/COUNTERPUNCH OPPORTUNITIES

Below are basic defensive move/counterpunch opportunities. Practice them slowly and then faster, until they "flow" without your having to think about them.

Left jab to your chin. Block with your right hand and step in with a left jab counter to the chin.

Parry with your right hand (photo, page 115). Counter with a left jab to the chin followed by a right cross thrown over the opposing (parried) left jab. (The right cross would be a "punch off the parry.")

Slip inside the punch. Potential counterpunches:

- A left jab to the chin followed by a straight right.
- A straight right to the chin.
- A right cross over your opponent's outstretched left.

Slip outside the punch. Potential counterpunches:

- A left to the body (see photo, page 117) followed by a right cross to the chin.
- A left hook to the chin.
- A right cross to the chin.
- A straight right or right uppercut to the body.

Left jab to your body. Block with your left forearm or elbow. Counter with a left jab to the chin, thrown over your opponent's (blocked) left.

Parry the blow by extending your right hand and pushing the blow downward. Counter with a left jab to the chin followed by a straight right.

120

Straight right to your chin. Block with your left hand. Potential counterpunches:

- Jab off the block, to your opponent's chin.
- Step in with a straight right to the chin.

Parry with your left hand, pushing the blow aside and downward. Potential counters:

- Jab off the parry, to your opponent's chin.
- Step in with a straight right to the chin, thrown over your opponent's (parried) right.

Slip inside the punch (photo, page 119) and simultaneously fire a straight right to your opponent's chin, followed by a left uppercut to his body.

Slip outside the punch and counter with a double hook: first to the body and then to the head.

Straight right to your body. Block with your left forearm or elbow. Counter with a jab off the block, to your opponent's chin.

Parry with your left hand and counter with a straight to the chin.

Left hook to your chin. Block with your right hand (photo, page 113). Potential counterpunches:

- A right to the chin off the block.
- A short left hook to the head.

Slip under the blow (so that it travels over your head). Counter with a right uppercut to the body and a left hook to the head.

With your chin "tucked" and your knees bent, step "inside" the arc of the blow so that it "wraps" around your neck. Counter with a short right to the chin.

Important: "Leaning back" to avoid punches is not recommended in general and is an especially unsafe way to attempt to avoid a left hook to the chin. Unless you're Muhammad Ali, when you lean back you'll get hit with the hook anyway, and you'll be off balance at the moment of impact. Defend against the hook by blocking it, slipping under it, or stepping inside it, as described above.

Left hook to your body. Block the blow with your right elbow and counter with a short right to the head.

Right uppercut to your chin or solar plexus. Parry with your right hand (photo, page 116) and counter with a left hook to the head, over your opponent's (parried) right hand. Again, don't hesitate with your counterpunch, or your opponent will hit you with a left hook to the head before you can launch your own. (Some boxers automatically launch a short left hook the instant they see a right uppercut coming.)

Parry with your left hand and counter with a straight right to the chin.

Left uppercut to your chin or solar plexus. Parry with your left hand and counter quickly with a straight right to the chin.

Parry with your right hand and launch a quick left hook to the chin.

CLINCHING

There are two reasons to clinch. The first is because he needs time to collect himself, due to fatigue or because his opponent has landed several consecutive blows and is likely to land more without effective resistance. The second is because his style is that of a brawling infighter who tries to "work the clinch" to his advantage.

The brawling style is generally frowned upon by boxing purists and is not recommended for the white-collar boxer: the "brawling" tendency becomes a ready crutch, one which mitigates the desire (and perceived need) to practice the more scientific fundamentals. Further, a brawling style can get the beginner hurt—a skillful opponent·knows how to step back and pick apart an inexperienced brawler. (It should be noted, however, that a brawling, infighting style *has* proven effective for some professionals: Mustafa Hamsho used it to become the world's number one middleweight contender. If not for Marvelous Marvin Hagler—one of the best contemporary champions—and his ability to "solve" Hamsho's style, Hamsho would certainly have become champion.) In summary, as a white-collar boxer you should use the clinch as a defensive move only, and you shouldn't need to use it too often.

How to clinch. Clinch by grabbing your opponent at the shoulders and moving your hands down his arms until you've successfully "wrapped" his arms in yours, making it difficult for him to punch effectively. Keep your head over one of your opponent's shoulders (but safely "tucked") throughout the clinch. Maintain the clinch by pressing close to your opponent until the referee (or your trainer) gives the "Break" command. Use your time in the clinch to breathe and find your center, so that you can resume the contest under control. Keep your hands up as you break. This will protect your head in case your opponent loses his and attempts (illegally) to "punch on the break."

Again, don't let your head "hang," especially when you're in a clinch with a crouching opponent: if he suddenly lifts his shoulder or head up, you'll be on the receiving end of a butt.

Although the clinch is presented above as a defensive move, it is all too often used offensively by boxers who try to get "cute." In the event that you find yourself in with a man who (illegally) likes to "hold and hit," there are two ways to defend. To prevent him from clinching in the first place, step back, set, and fire straight punch combinations to his head as he attempts to "wrap" you. If you're in a clinch and want to get out, "punch out," by firing uppercuts to the midsection, aiming for the solar plexus. This will "back up" your opponent and cause his head to hang and his hands to drop—so that you can easily step forward and land a hook to his chin.

COVERING UP

If you need to "cover up," it means you're in over your head: not only can't you mount an attack or defend and counterpunch; you can't even manage to clinch. A good trainer keeps you out of these situations, by matching you carefully and watching you closely when you spar. If he notices that you simply can't cope, he'll immediately demand that your opponent "lighten up." If you're feeling overwhelmed and your trainer isn't intervening quickly enough for your health, simply call "time," walk over to your trainer, and tell him to ask your opponent to "work" with you. If you resume activity and find that you're still unable to cope, simply get out of the ring and tell your trainer to match you more carefully the next time—or you'll find another trainer.

During many years of periodic sparring, I was forced to "cover up" only once, and that situation was quickly remedied by Al Gavin. To help prepare me for an upcoming Golden Gloves match, Al put me in with a professional lightweight contender who happened to be training at the Gramercy. I had sparred with professionals many times before—in every case they "went easy," recognizing the unwritten boxing law that "the sparring session is for the man with the least experience." Maybe my professional opponent was having a bad day; maybe he was just a nasty sonofabitch. At any rate, he completely overwhelmed me: I "covered up" by hunching my shoulders forward and tucking my chin, drawing my hands and elbows in close, and going into a protective "shell" so that the majority of his punches hit my elbows and gloves. Although I wasn't getting hurt, I clearly couldn't counterpunch from this position, and I knew it was just a matter of time until one of his many blows "got through." Al was right on top of the situation. After only a few seconds under my opponent's barrage, I heard Al admonish him sharply. He immediately backed away and apologized. He "played defense" from that point on, letting me get my punches off (he slipped nearly all of them) and throwing an occasional jab or light counterpunch, as if to politely "point out" the openings he saw.

DEVELOPING YOUR PERSONAL BOXING STYLE

You should strive to be a *complete* boxer, with the ability to jab and move, fight inside, defend, and counterpunch. At the same time, it's important to develop a personal boxing "style" that makes the most of your physical advantages. The majority of pugilists can be loosely categorized as "boxers," infighters, or counterpunchers. A smaller but still significant portion fall between categories. Finally, a special few transcend them altogether—for example, Sugar Ray Robinson, who could simply do it all.

The Three Basic Styles

Each of the three basic boxing styles is discussed below. Consider each carefully as you work to perfect your personal boxing style.

If you're tall for your weight and enjoy a reach advantage, you'll benefit from a jabbing, "boxing" style. This calls for quick hands; specifically a fast and accurate jab and double jab, quick and graceful ring movement, and a keen sense of "distance."

Your operating philosophy as a "boxer" can be reduced to one sentence: Exploit your reach advantage. Specifically, you should box with the clear recognition that it's in your overriding interest to "make the fight" from that precise and ideal distance where your punches can reach your opponent, but his can't reach you. You should generally circle in the direction of your jabbing hand, firing the jab frequently in order to measure your opponent and maintain the aforementioned "ideal distance," pile up points, set up combinations, and stay away from trouble. Step forward with a crisp combination the moment you sense that your jab (or series of jabs) has your opponent confused, fatigued, or dazed. After you've thrown your combination, quickly "get out" of your opponent's range. Evaluate the situation as you jab and circle once more: If it feels right, step in with another combination.

Stay out of the corners, where your reach advantage (and jab) are nullified, and you're more easily hit. If your opponent succeeds in getting inside your jab, "tie him up" until the referee breaks you; then resume your jab-and-circle pattern. Don't get suckered into trading punches on the inside. This isn't your kind of fight; your reach advantage is rendered useless.

THE INFIGHTER

If you're short for your weight and at a reach disadvantage, you'll need to adopt an "infighting" style. This calls for the stamina and persistence necessary to force the action, and the quickness needed to "cut the ring," slip punches, and throw effective combinations once you're "inside."

As an infighter, your operating philosophy can be summed up in four words: get inside and punch. It is on the inside that you can nullify your opponent's reach advantage and land the telling combinations to wear him down. In order to get inside, you'll first need to "cut the ring." "Cutting the ring" is best defined by example. If your opponent circles to his left (your right), "cut him off" by moving forward and to your right, and vice-versa. Your "cut-off" opponent has several options, none of which are to his advantage:

He can hold his ground and try to "slug it out" at close range. However, from this (shorter) distance his reach advantage is negated. What's more, his longer arms can actually do him a disservice: From in close, they necessarily won't be fully extended at impact. This minimizes the power of his straight punches. Additionally, many less experienced "boxers" have a tendency to "wrap" their left hook (around the back of your neck) when forced to launch it from in close.

He can change direction, in which case you should too, until he's literally "cornered" and forced to fight "your kind of fight."

He can try to clinch, by "wrapping" his arms around yours. In this case you should fire straight-punch combinations to his head as he steps forward. This will cause him to raise his hands defensively, creating openings for body shots and ultimately enabling you to sustain the in-close type of fight which is your forte.

After you've cut the ring, don't just "walk in" as if to announce "Here I am," or you'll get nailed. If your opponent punches, slip the oncoming blow as you step inside. If he hesitates, step inside behind your left jab. Once you're inside, you've got to punch, hard and in combination, or else the energy you expended to get there is simply wasted. *(Note:* Many so-called infighters work hard to get inside and then just "lay there." They lean on their opponent and let him clinch, as if getting inside is alone enough to win the contest. It isn't. What matters is not aggression, but *meaningful* aggression.)

THE COUNTERPUNCHER

It's not without some hesitation that counterpunchers are put into a separate category. After all, "boxers" and infighters both rely heavily on counterpunching, and "counterpunchers" can usually "box" and/or infight. At the same time, there is a small but noteworthy group of boxers (Wilfred Benitez heads the list) whose bread and butter is effective counterpunching.

Effective counterpunchers are enigmatic: they have great quickness, but their style usually slows the overall pace of a match. They

126

are cool and calculating as they study their opponent for tendencies and patterns, yet are able to improvise like the most impassioned jazz player if an unexpected opening suddenly presents itself. Supremely confident, their operating philosophy goes something like: "I'm going to let you try to hit me first. Not only will you miss, you'll leave yourself open as you do. And then I'm going to hit you, hard and in combination."

The counterpuncher is usually at least as tall as his opponent, though not necessarily as tall as "boxer" types. He usually fights at a middle distance: far enough away so that he isn't easily hit or forced to punch, yet close enough so that he can easily step or slip inside. He lets his opponent press the action, jabbing periodically and maintaining this "middle" distance until the time is right.

Before you can call yourself a "counterpuncher," your defensive skills of course need to be excellent: you should be completely at ease with slipping, and countering off the slip. You should have developed your ability to feint—not just with your hands, but with your shoulders, legs, and even your eyes. And you should have the quickness (and confidence) to successfully *draw* punches, by lowering a hand on purpose and then quickly slipping the "drawn" blow and firing an effective counterpunch.

As if the above-required skills weren't enough, there's more: you've got to be patient, in order to give your opponent a chance to make the very mistakes that you hope to counter. (This is difficult for beginning boxers, who tend to feel uncomfortable if they're not "doing something.") Finally, you've got to counter in combination, to make the most of every opportunity.

Counterpunching is in my opinion the most difficult style for the beginning boxer to master. My recommendation is to first adopt a "boxing" or infighting style (whichever is appropriate for you), and develop your counterpunching skills within that style. As you gain experience and confidence in your counterpunching, it can come to play an increasingly important role in your personal boxing style.

ADDITIONAL CONSIDERATIONS

Evaluate yourself objectively. Be realistic about your strengths, weaknesses, and physical characteristics. If you're short and stocky, it's foolish to attempt to box from a distance, even if you've always dreamed of floating like a butterfly. If you're tall and thin, an infighting style is not in your interest. And if you're the worst Ping-Pong player you know, it's probably not wise to embrace the reaction-oriented style of a counterpuncher (at least not without lots of practice).

Adapt your style to meet the opponent and situation. Your style is the starting point for the development of your ring strategy, but it should not be that strategy in itself. You'll need to make modifications, sometimes subtle ones, which recognize your opponent's style and tendencies, as well as what you have reason to believe he thinks you're going to do.

Example: You're an infighter who's known to work to set up his left hook. You're fighting a counterpuncher. While you might normally get inside by stepping in behind your left jab or slipping past oncoming punches, you can expect these tactics to be less effective now: your counterpunching opponent wants you to throw left leads so he has something to counter. At the same time, he'll throw a minimum number of leads himself, so that you'll have nothing to slip. Recognizing this situation, you should feign punches frequently as you move to cut him off. This will draw his counterpunches (to the leads you never threw). You can then slip inside, past his (non-)counterpunches. Once inside, feign the left hook frequently and instead throw straight rights. By emphasizing feints and your straight right (instead of the expected lead lefts and left hook), you'll have adapted your infighting style to meet the circumstance. (More on boxing strategy in Chapter Five.)

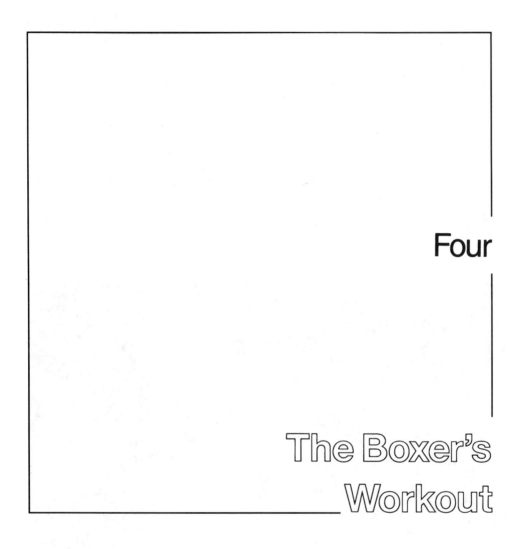

Four

The Boxer's Workout

Once you've completed your preconditioning period and are familiar with the essential physical moves described in the previous chapter, you're ready to begin regular Boxer's Workouts.

The following four key points are worth reiterating:

A gradual approach is the best approach. Start with easier Boxer's Workouts, concentrating primarily on technique. Increase the duration and intensity of your Boxer's Workouts only when you're fully ready. Remember not to punch too hard too soon.

A "hard day/easy day" schedule will improve your performance and minimize the risk of injury. Again, a prototype schedule calls for (harder) Boxer's Workouts three times per week, with (easier) roadwork on the off days, and one day of complete rest.

Drink water before, during, and after your workouts. Hydrate about a half hour before every Boxer's Workout. (Drink at least a pint of water.) Drink a moderate amount of water at least every two rounds. On especially warm days, drink a small amount of water before every round.

Concentrate on being relaxed. Discipline yourself to stay on center. Give your full attention to the task at hand. Visualize your opponent as you perform your moves with no wasted motion. Breathe.

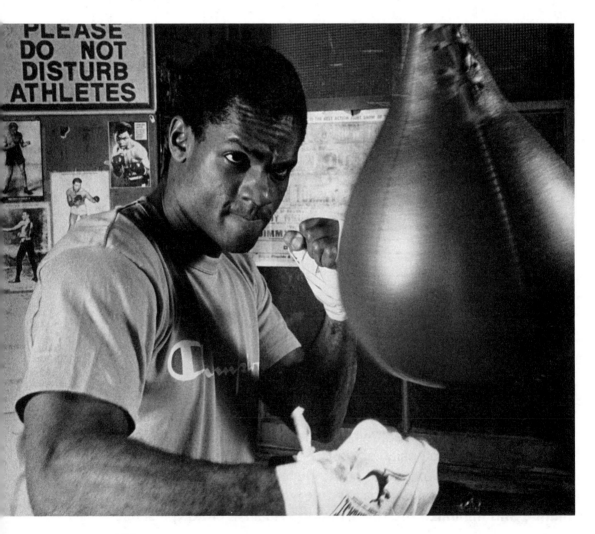

Exercises should be performed in the order below, with your effort building to a crescendo on the heavy bag.

1. Warmup and stretches
2. Mirror training
3. Shadowboxing
4. Heavy bag
5. Speed bag
6. Double-end bag (optional)
7. Jump rope
8. Stomach exercises: sit-ups and crunches standard, medicine ball optional

INTENSITY AND DURATION

In the sequence above, the first exercise (warm-up and stretches) and the last (stomach exercises) take about five minutes each. (Stomach exercises will take a bit longer if you choose to include optional work on the medicine ball.) The exercises in between are performed by the "round." By varying the number of rounds per exercise and the length of each round, you can do the Boxer's Workout at each of three basic workout levels. There's one minute of "rest" between rounds, regardless of your workout level.

WORKOUT LEVEL	WORKOUT LOCATION	NUMBER OF ROUNDS PER EXERCISE*	MINUTES PER ROUND	TOTAL "WORKING" MINUTES† (APPROX.)
Beginning (6 Weeks)	Home or Fitness Club (Only)	2	2	30
Moderate (6 Weeks)	Home, Fitness Club, or Boxing Gym	2	3	40
Intensive	Home, Fitness Club, or Boxing Gym	3	3	55

*Exercises done by the round include mirror training, shadowboxing, heavy bag, speed bag, double-end bag (optional), and jump rope.

†Excludes "rest" minutes between rounds and any time you might spend on the double-end bag or medicine ball, which are optional.

Important: In a boxing gym, the bell is timed to sound according to three minutes of work/one minute of rest schedule, reflecting the three minutes of boxing/one minute of rest pace of a professional boxing match. If you choose from the outset to do your Boxer's Workouts in a boxing gym, you'll necessarily be working out at this three-minute round length—that is, at the "moderate" level. Compensate—and protect yourself from overstress and injury—by extending your moderate-level training period to twelve weeks and adopting an especially easy pace during your first six weeks.

If you choose to do your Boxer's Workouts at home or fitness club, you'll be able to shorten your rounds to two minutes during your "Beginning" period. Don't feel bashful about this. Two-minute rounds are used in most amateur contests, and two minutes can seem like two hours when you're firing combinations at the heavy bag.

Use a stopwatch or runner's watch to time yourself at home or at a fitness club. Eventually you'll come to know almost exactly how long two (and then three) minutes are, and will need to look at your watch only occasionally.

For each exercise in the circuit, start slowly and work up to greatest intensity toward the middle of the round. During the "rest" minute, breathe deeply and "shake out" your arms as you walk around or bounce lightly on the balls of your feet. "Center" yourself before starting the next round.

Although the component exercises are of course presented separately, I encourage you to view your workout as a whole; with each exercise flowing smoothly into the next and with you "getting warmer" as you go.

WARMUP AND STRETCHES

Perform the following exercises in order:

Find your center. Stand in front of the mirror. Begin to breathe deeply from your belly. As you breathe, let go of any tightness in your shoulders and let your arms hang. Clear your mind of extraneous thoughts. Forget about your job, about any of the boxers around you, about any onlookers. Relax into that private space where you can concentrate fully.

Boxer's bounce. With your weight on the balls of your feet and your arms still hanging, bounce gently in place. Shift your weight from one foot to the other, with your feet barely leaving the floor. Continue this easy bounce for about two minutes. Feel your pulse begin to rise as your heart pumps the extra blood your muscles need in order to stretch easily and safely.

Forward hang. Starting from the top of your head, slowly hang forward, vertebra by vertebra, until you're fully bent at the waist with your arms dangling in front of you. Your knees should be bent slightly. Hold the fully bent position for three slow, deep breaths. Don't rock, bounce, or try to touch your toes. Just "hang" forward and breathe. You'll feel your lower back and hamstrings begin to loosen. Come up very slowly, vertebra by vertebra, and go into gentle neck rolls, slowly moving your head from side to side.

Trunk stretch (photo, page 134). With feet apart as shown, place the palm of your right hand behind your head such that the inside of your right biceps, elbow, and forearm face forward. Slowly bend left from the waist, until you begin to feel resistance in the oblique muscles on the right side of your waist. As you bend, be sure to keep your elbow up and on the same plane as your forehead, as shown. (There's a tendency to let your elbow fall forward.) Hold the fully bent position for three deep breaths; then release and come up slowly. Repeat the exercise in the alternate direction.

Groin stretch (photo, page 135). With your feet wide apart as shown, slowly and carefully begin to bend your right knee, while your left knee remains straight. Be aware of your "center" as you go into the stretch—this will help you to stay on balance. As you bend your right knee farther, place your arms as shown for added support and balance. Bend your knee until you feel resistance in your inner thigh (adductor) muscles. Hold this position for three deep breaths; then release. Repeat the exercise in the alternate direction.

Arm circles (photo, page 136). With your feet comfortably apart, raise your hands to shoulder level, with your elbows straight, as shown. With your palms facing upward, do thirty small arm circles in the backward direction. For maximum benefit, be sure to get your shoulders into the motion. After you've completed your backward

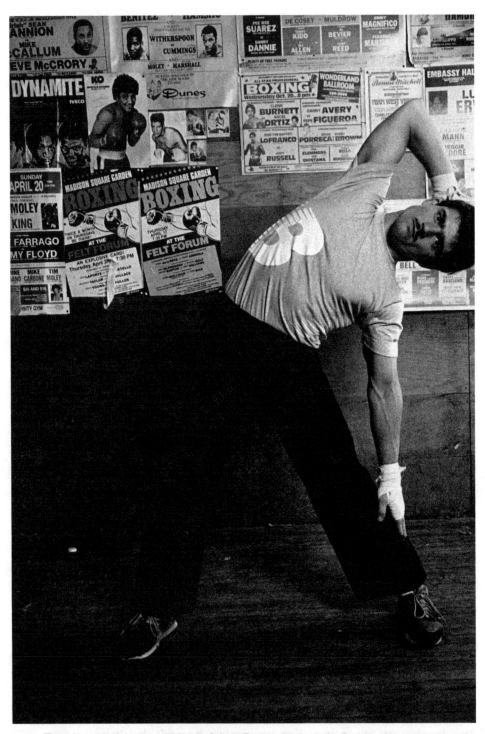

*Trunk stretch: performed by Robert Jaeckel, programmer ana-
lyst, Cologne Life Reinsurance Company.*

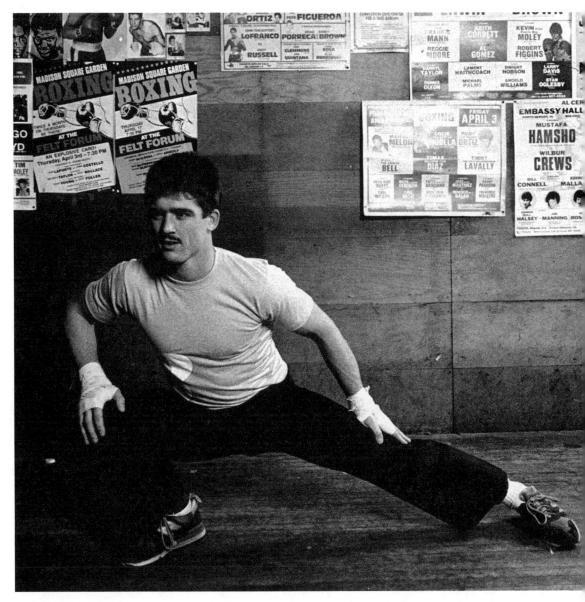

Groin stretch.

arm circles, flip your palms so they face the floor and do thirty small arm circles in the forward direction.

Windmill (photo, page 137). Think of these as larger arm circles, important to more fully loosen your shoulder and back muscles. With your elbows straight and palms upward, do thirty windmills in the backward direction. Flip your palms; then do thirty windmills in

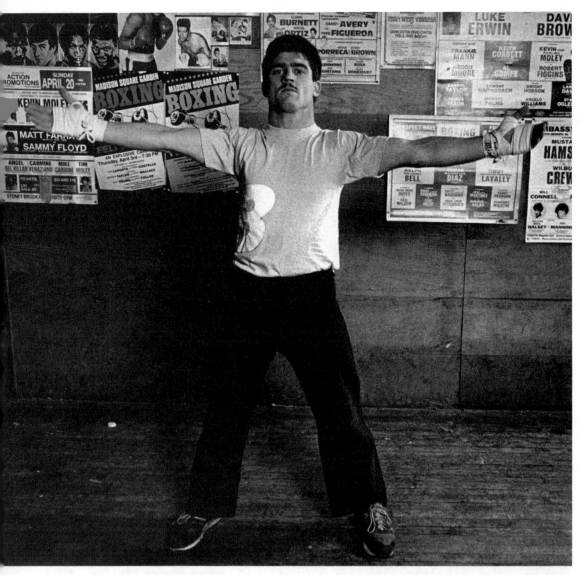

Arm circles.

the forward direction. Start the motion slowly and increase the speed as you go, up to a moderate level.

IMPORTANT POINTS TO REMEMBER

Always warm up before you stretch, with the Boxer's Bounce or some other similar exercise. Don't stretch when you're completely cold—there's insufficient blood in your muscles to provide

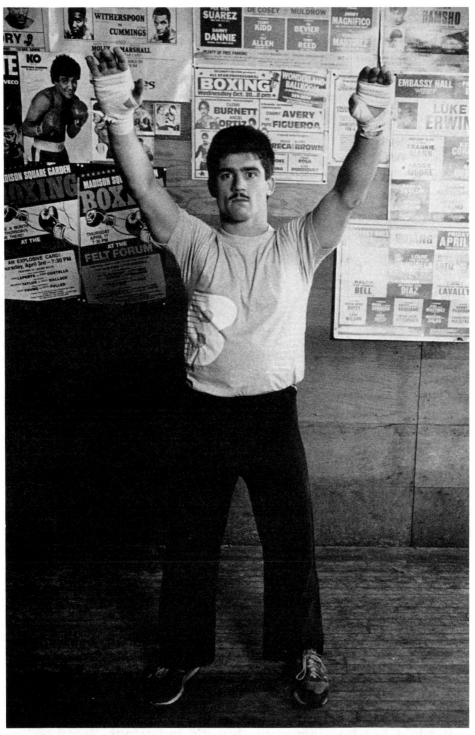

Windmill.

the added oxygen they need to exercise. In other words, don't just put on your sweats and drop into an extra-deep groin stretch—you may not be able to stand up again.

Stretching isn't competitive. Don't worry about how far you can or can't stretch compared to others. Stretch only to your point of resistance, hold for three deep breaths, then release. Drop any self-flagellating notions like "stretching beyond the pain"—they'll leave you with nothing but pulled muscles.

Always go in and out of a stretch very gently. Stretch your muscles with the sensitivity and respect they deserve. They'll pay you back by performing better for you through your workout.

Breathe as you stretch. This helps you to relax and of course releases carbon dioxide, the toxic by-product of the very muscles you're working.

MIRROR TRAINING

Assume your classic stance in front of the mirror. Get relatively close. There should be about a foot of air between you and the glass when your left jab is fully extended. Check your stance. Do you feel on balance? Are your legs comfortably apart and your hands properly positioned? Are you sideways toward your opponent with your chin tucked?

As the round begins, start slowly. The emphasis is on technique rather than speed or force. First throw your straight punches, in slow motion. Get the mechanics correct. When you're comfortable with how your straight punches look and feel, work in your uppercut and hook. Envision your opponent in front of you as you practice your defensive moves.

Rehearse your combinations, starting with the basic one-two and working up to the more advanced combinations. Remember to work feints into your combinations. Increase your speed and intensity as you get warmer, but don't hesitate to revert to slow motion if something doesn't look or feel right.

IMPORTANT POINTS TO REMEMBER

It might not be glamorous, but it's important. Some boxers give mirror training the back of their hand, or omit it altogether be-

138

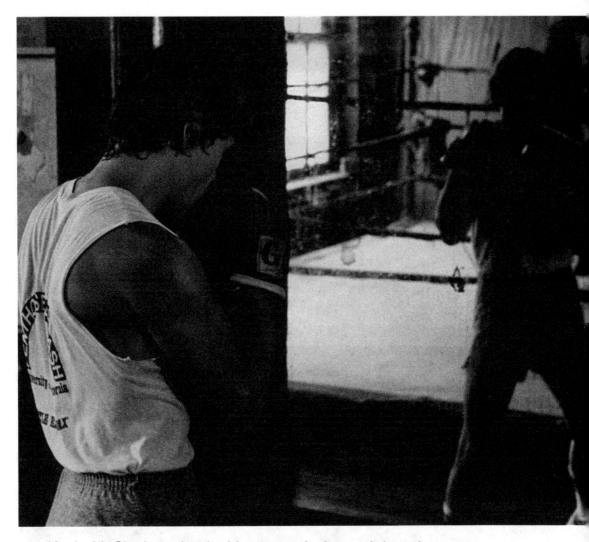

Kevin McCloskey checks his stance in front of the mirror . . .

cause it's not as macho or exciting as actually hitting something. The better boxers, however, give mirror training the time and importance it deserves. They know that it sets the tone for the rest of their workout, and that if their technique isn't correct in front of the mirror—where they can see it—it won't be right on the heavy bag or in the ring.

Use the mirror as an easy reference tool. If you're shadowboxing in the ring or working on the heavy bag and a punch or move

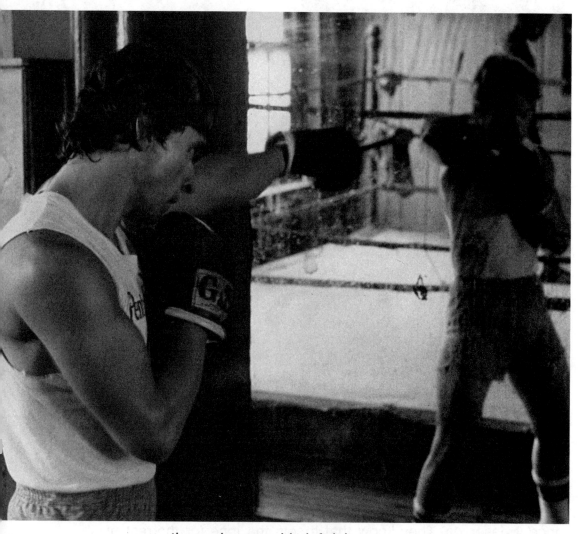

. . . then rehearses his left jab . . .

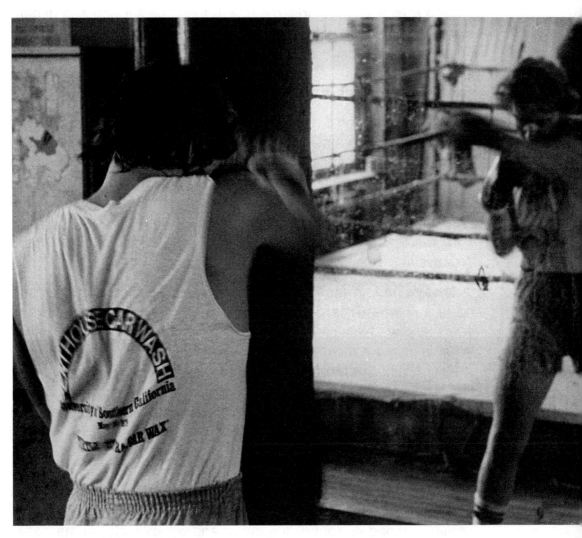

. . . *and his straight right.*

seems awkward or incorrect, check the move on the mirror during your "rest" minute.

SHADOWBOXING

Step into the ring. Observe how it feels: its surface and dimensions. Imagine your opponent in front of you as you begin to move. Feel your pulse quicken as you start to put it all together: hand speed and footwork, offense and defense.

Move and punch as you would during a match:

- If you've adopted a "boxing" style, jab and move in concentric circles. (Imagine a pebble falling into a pool.) Step in and out with specific combinations.
- If you're an infighter, move forward and sideways behind your left jab as you "cut off" your "boxer" opponent. Throw combinations as you get inside.
- To develop counterpunching skills, be sure to work feints and draws into your movement.

Always have a mental picture of your opponent. Know where he is and what he's doing. See his punches coming at you, and yours landing. How did he react to the combination you just threw? What is his next move? What should yours be?

Recognize the length of a round. Shadowboxing provides your first real taste of just how long three minutes is. Pace yourself accordingly. At the end of the round, you should be breathing hard but ready for more.

IMPORTANT POINTS TO REMEMBER

Shadowboxing should always be purposeful. It serves as a proving ground for the combinations and moves you've slowly and carefully honed in front of the mirror and will execute on the heavy bag and during any sparring. It's not "bouncing around," or "loosening up."

Shadowbox slowly when necessary. If a specific combination is giving you trouble, isolate and shadowbox through it in slow motion before resuming your more rigorous overall pace.

142

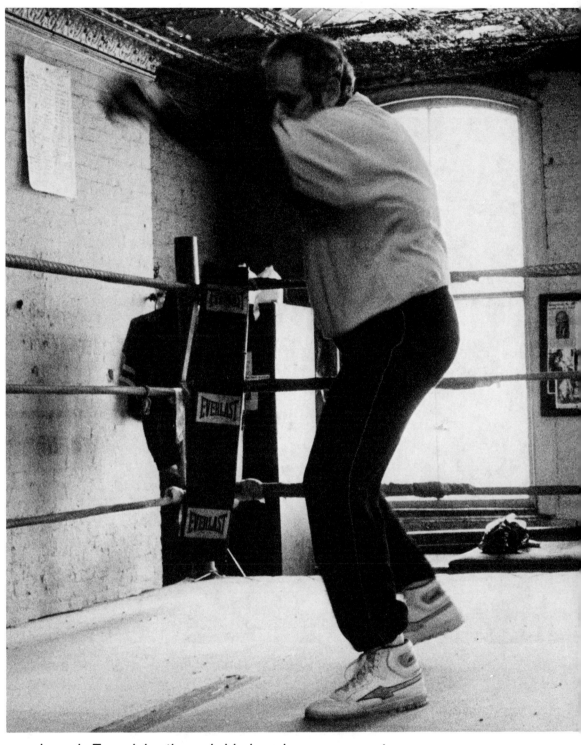

Joseph Egan jabs through his imaginary opponent.

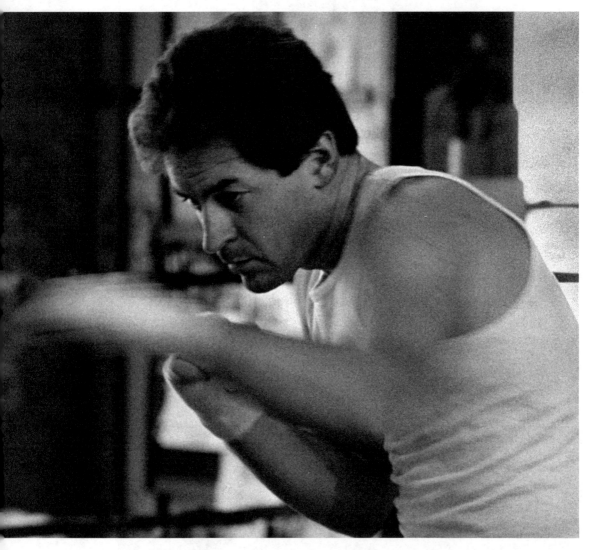

Note the concentration as Ray Ginther throws a left and a straight right. Shadowboxing should always be purposeful.

144

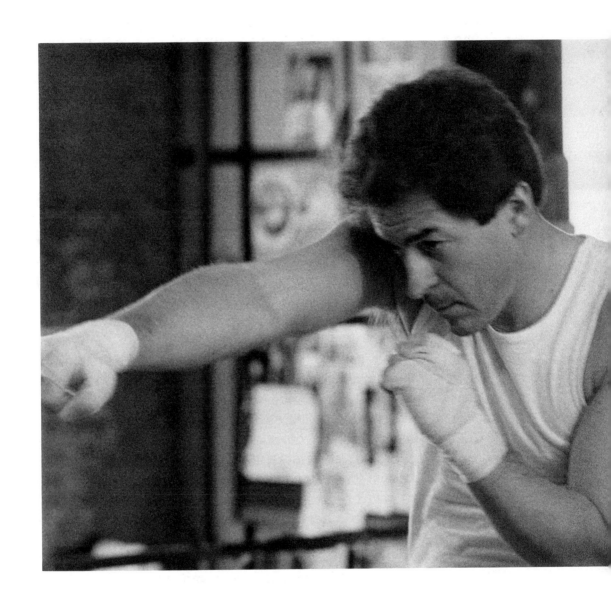

There is your opponent, big and tough. You can see his face right on the surface of the bag. You honed your technique in front of the mirror. You worked on it some more as you stepped up your pace during shadowboxing. Now slip on your striking mitts and turn that technique into power.

Begin by measuring your distance. For straight punches, position yourself so that your punching arm will be fully extended at the moment of impact. Your hook and uppercut should of course be launched from in close.

As you prepare to launch a punch, visualize it being delivered so correctly that it breaks the bag in two. Bring your power up from the balls of your feet, focus it in your fist, and deliver it *through* the bag.

Work on your straight punches first, then on your hook and uppercut. Practice each punch until you're satisfied that it's mechanically correct and powerful. When you land a blow correctly, you actually *feel* the power. You'll eventually come to know and strive for that "right feeling" with every punch.

When you're comfortable with your individual punches, start putting together combinations. This can be difficult. Component punches must come in rapid-fire succession, yet each must have your full force behind it, delivered through the bag. Practice.

Control the bag the way you would control your opponent. Move and punch according to your style. If you're a boxer, jab and double-jab as you circle in the direction of your jabbing hand. Step in with crisp combinations off the jab; then step out and circle again. If you're an infighter, go in behind your jab and throw head-body combinations.

There is greater intensity during this exercise. Your heart rate is higher than at any other point during the workout.

IMPORTANT POINTS TO REMEMBER

Greater power comes largely through better technique. The most effective way to maximize your power is to perfect your punching mechanics.

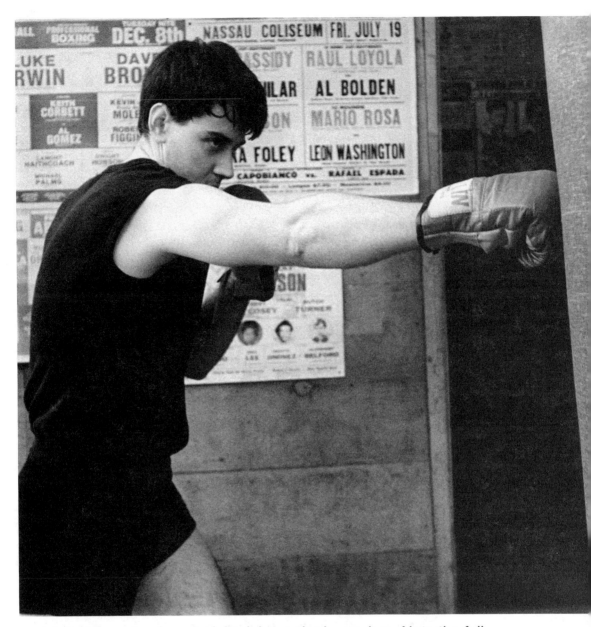

John Haran lands a straight right on the heavy bag. Note the full extension of his punching arm at impact.

Punch—don't "push." Punches are powerful—"pushes" aren't. If your punch reaches the bag before it's supposed to, the result is a slow, ineffective "push." *Remember:* Your punching arm should be

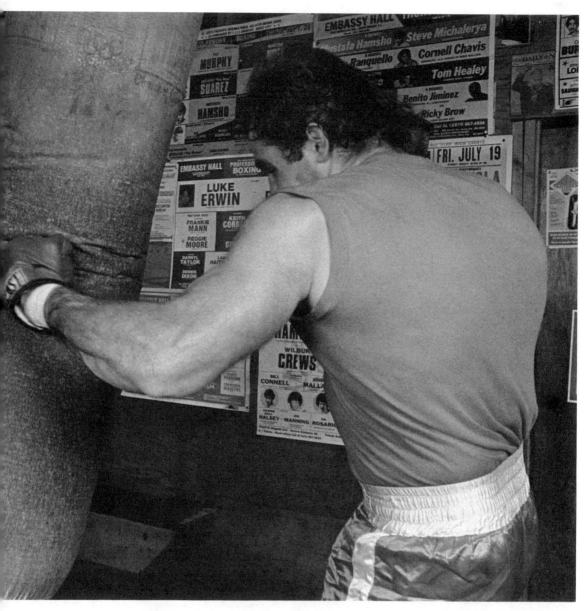

Martin Snow lands a left hook from in close.

fully extended at impact for straight punches, and your hook and uppercut should be well along their trajectory as they strike the bag.

Keep your wrists straight at all times. Remember to think of your wrist and fist as one unit. This will minimize the chance of wrist injuries.

148

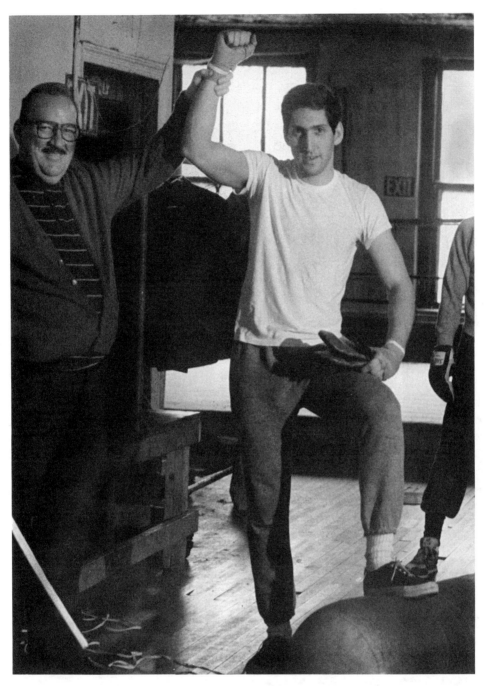

Control the heavy bag the way you would control your opponent. Here: Bob Jackson congratulates Spenser Alpern, president of Spenser Jeremy Dress, Inc., New York, after Spenser felled the heavy bag with a particularly devastating combination.

149

Hand speed and coordination are vital to effective combination punching. The speed bag helps you develop them. It also builds your arm and shoulder strength. It isn't easy to keep your hands up and maintain a continuous punching rhythm for a full three minutes.

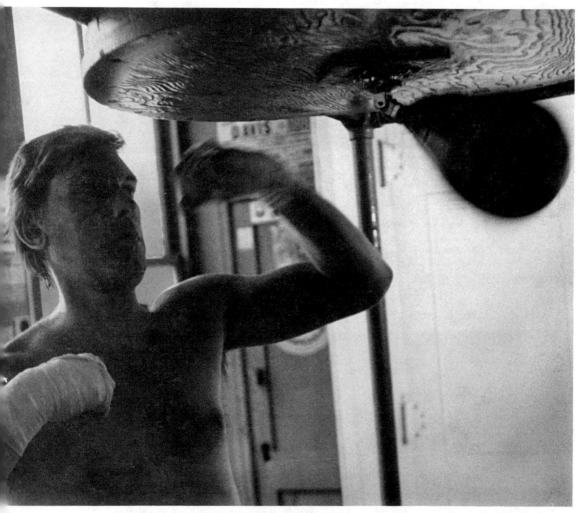

Stay focused on your rhythm. Robert Elsasser, senior account manager for the Codex Corporation, works on the speed bag.

Start with a larger bag, for the simple reason that these move slower. (You'll get better with practice and will eventually "move down" to a smaller, quicker bag.)

Some boxers wear their striking mitts for speed bag work; others (including the author) don't. My advice is to try it without mitts first, but to slip them on quickly if you feel any irritation.

Stand directly in front of the bag. (This contrasts with the classic stance, which has you sideways toward your opponent.) Distribute your weight equally on the balls of your feet, without rising up on your toes. The bag should be set at eye level.

The standard punching rhythm has four beats: (1) strike the bag, (2) the bag hits the far part of the platform, (3) the bag hits the near part of the platform, (4) the bag hits the far part of platform again—and comes back toward you to be struck once more. Allow two strikes per hand before alternating: the first strike with the front of your fist, the second with the back.

At the outset, strive to maintain a slow, steady rhythm. If your rhythm is broken, quickly steady the bag before you start again. Keep your hands up. If you drop a hand between strikes, it's almost impossible to raise it again in time to hold your rhythm.

Once you're able to hold a moderate rhythm for an entire round, you might intersperse surges of quicker punching, circle the bag as you strike it, or switch hands with every strike. As the end of the round approaches, your shoulders will be screaming and you'll be breathing hard. Stay focused on your rhythm.

IMPORTANT POINTS TO REMEMBER

Don't be intimidated. Experienced pros turn speed bag work into artistry. They work on "peanut" bags, which move much too quickly for the beginner. They vary their punches and punching rhythm. They even strike the bag with their elbows periodically. As impressive as the pros might be, remember that they started with the same objective as you: to hold a basic punching rhythm on a larger speed bag for an entire round.

"Slow down" your bag if necessary. If you're having a particularly difficult time establishing a rhythm, consider slowing down your bag by underinflating it. As you feel ready to handle greater speed, you can increase the amount of air in the bag.

DOUBLE-END BAG (OPTIONAL)

The ability to slip a punch and then land an effective counterpunch coming out of the slip is an important sign of a better boxer. Once you've become comfortable with slipping by practicing it in front of the mirror, during shadowboxing, and during your work on the heavy bag, you might want to hone this skill further by spending a couple of rounds on the double-end bag. As described earlier, this apparatus consists of a ball, about the size of a soccer ball, suspended at eye level by elastic ropes at either end. You strike the ball, slip it as it travels back toward you, and then launch your next punch so that it strikes the ball flush. (The purpose and method of slipping is described on pages 116–120.)

Put your striking mitts on and stand at arm's length from the ball. Start slowly. Throw light, straight punches without stepping in as you punch. The ball will, of course, snap back toward your head, but it will fall an inch or two short of striking you. Throw several punches from this distance, without stepping in. Follow the ball back toward you each time, without squinting, tightening up, or engaging in any other anxiety that might cause you to take your eye off the ball. The idea is for you to get used to seeing something *come at* you, while you get a feel for the amount of play in the ball.

After you're familiar with how the ball responds to your punches, begin to step into each punch and then slip the ball as it snaps back toward you. The ball should pass over either shoulder. At first, your slips will be exaggerated. Gradually, you'll come to slip more efficiently, moving your head just enough to avoid the ball and no more. Your slip should serve as the first (launching) part of your counterpunch, which should strike the bag as it springs toward you a second time. Practice each of the major combinations presented earlier.

JUMP ROPE

The jump rope improves cardiovascular efficiency and coordination. While jumping rope has recently been rediscovered as an ex-

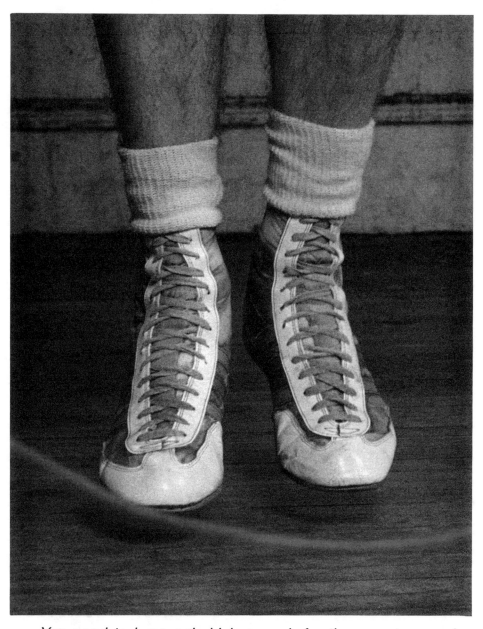

You need to jump only high enough for the rope to pass be-neath your feet.

cellent total body exercise in its own right, the rope has been a part of the boxer's routine for years.

Start by making sure your rope is the correct length. (Because most manufacturers adopt a "one size fits all" philosophy, a new jump rope is often too long.) Stand on the rope with both feet; then pull up on the handles. The top of the handles should be level with your armpits. Shorten the rope by knotting it close to the handles.

Your movement should be easy and economical. The initial goal is to establish a steady rhythm and maintain it for an entire round. Your weight is on the balls of your feet. Bend your knees slightly to help absorb impact and to power subsequent jumps. Rotate the rope primarily with your wrists, keeping your elbows close to your body. Don't jump unnecessarily high! This is the most common beginner's mistake, one which wastes energy and makes it impossible to establish a smooth, easy rhythm. At first, skip with both feet. Eventually you'll learn to skip one foot at a time.

As you get better on the rope, you'll be able to vary the action; always easily able to fall back to a moderate, regular pace. Intersperse bursts of quicker jumping. Step forward and backward, and from side to side—eventually you'll be able to make a circle. Run in place as you jump. Insert double skips, with the rope passing underfoot twice per jump.

The finish should leave you winded but loose.

IMPORTANT POINTS TO REMEMBER

Listen to your own tune. Try not to look at other rope skippers as you're trying to skip yourself—they're likely to throw you off rhythm. Concentrate fully on establishing and maintaining your own pace.

Don't make it harder than it needs to be. Beginners tend to grimace, tighten up, jump rigidly, and jump too high. Relax. We're only jumping rope.

STOMACH EXERCISES

Boxers inevitably get hit with body blows—their stomach muscles must be able to withstand the impact. The following basic exercises are used by boxers everywhere to help toughen abdominal muscles:

Bent-knee sit-ups (right). These exercise the lower abdominals. Lie flat on your back, with your hands behind your head and your knees bent. Exhale as you come up slowly, until the inside

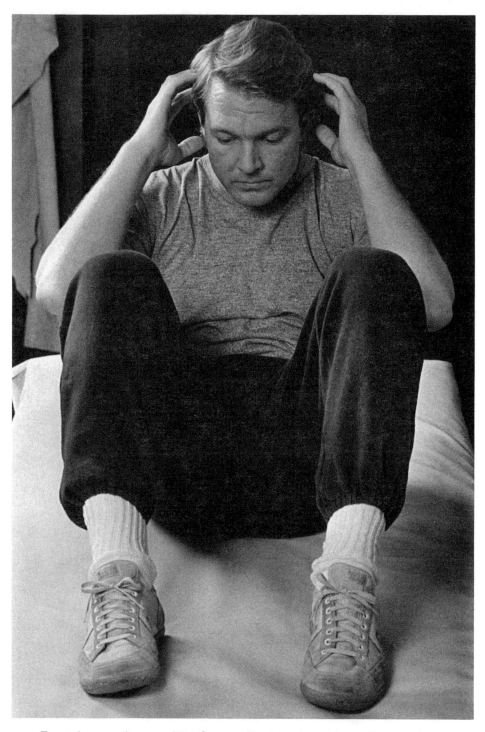

Bent-knee sit-ups: W. Gregg Porter does bent-knee sit-ups to work his lower abdominals.

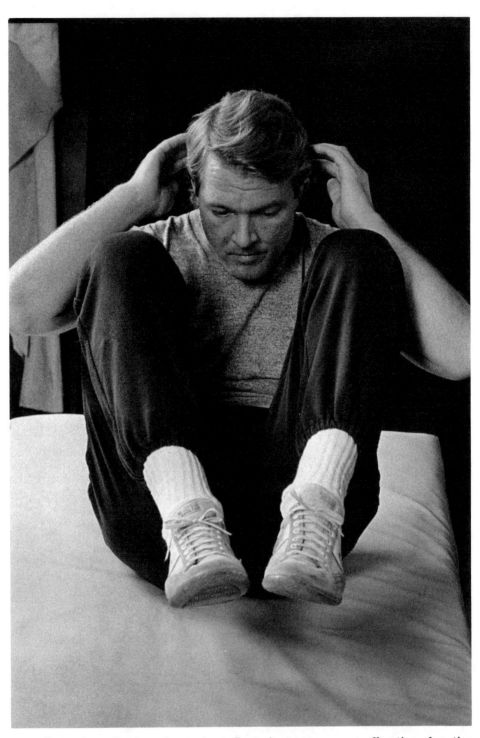

Crunches feel awkward at first, but are very effective for the upper abdominals.

of your elbows meets the outside of your knees. Start with two slow sets of twenty, allowing thirty seconds of rest in between the sets.

Crunches (left). These feel awkward at first, but are very effective for the upper abdominals. Again lie flat on your back, with your hands behind your head and your knees bent. Come up into the crunch position by slowly (but simultaneously) raising your knees and bringing your elbows up until they meet the outside of your knees (as shown). Be sure to exhale as you come up into the crunch position. Start with two slow sets of twenty, with thirty seconds of rest in between sets.

IMPORTANT POINTS TO REMEMBER

Slower is better. Don't rush through your repetitions. Slower reps help insure that your movement is technically correct, reduce the sudden jerks that can cause strains, and have you hold each muscle contraction longer.

Don't come up too far. If you bring your elbows too far forward, you reduce the amount of work being performed by your abdominals and instead begin using—and possibly straining—your lower back.

The Medicine Ball (Optional)

Work on the medicine ball is optional but recommended. However, don't consider adding the medicine ball to your stomach regimen until you can comfortably perform each of the exercises above.

Medicine ball work comes out of a simple principle embraced by many boxing trainers, especially the oldtimers. The best way to prepare yourself to absorb blows to the stomach is to absorb blows to the stomach. There are two basic ways to use the medicine ball:

MEDICINE BALL CATCH

This exercise calls for you to "play catch" with a partner who is of roughly equal weight. If you work out in a boxing gym or fitness club, a partner is, of course, easier to find than if you work out at home. (If a partner is unavailable, substitute the solo medicine ball work described below.) If you are fortunate enough to find a steady and willing partner, you'll both quickly come to realize that medicine ball

157

catch can be even more fun than Lazer Tag. Start by facing each other, about an arm's length apart.

To launch the medicine ball, hold the ball at either side, just above your navel. Using both hands, "push" (rather than "throw") the ball into your partner. Exhale deeply as you push. The ball should make contact with your partner just above his navel, just as your arms reach full extension. Be sure to aim the ball correctly. If you place it too high, you'll be endangering your partner's ribs; too low, and you'll make an enemy forever. Make your first few "pushes" very easy, and increase the force only as your partner tells you to do so.

To receive the medicine ball, stand with your arms at your sides and tense your abdominals as the ball comes toward you. Exhale as you absorb the full force of the ball with your abdominals, and then grasp the ball on either side as it begins to drop. Inhale deeply, and then exhale deeply as you push the ball back toward your partner.

SOLO WORK ON THE MEDICINE BALL

Lie flat on your back, with your knees bent. Rest the medicine ball on the area just above your navel. Steady the ball by grasping it on either side. Gently toss the ball a few inches straight up into the air, so that it will land on exactly the same spot from which it was launched. Tense your abdominals and exhale as the ball strikes; then grasp it at either side and toss it up once again. Increase the height of your tosses only as you feel ready to absorb the increased force.

When you can do the above exercise easily (by this time your abdominals will be as tough as boilerplate), you might consider increasing the frequency of strikes without compromising the force, by doing the following: Starting from exactly the same position as above, lift the ball directly over your abdomen and then forcefully throw it back into the same spot. Tense your abdominals and exhale as the ball strikes; then quickly repeat the exercise.

A brief note on cooldown. After you've finished your stomach exercises, don't rush straight into the shower. Take a few deep breaths from your belly, savor your workout, and let your pulse return to normal before you call it a day.

TAKING IT ON THE ROAD

There's no need to lose your edge on business trips. A modified Boxer's Workout will help keep you sharp until you return home. Except for the heavy bag and speed bag, you can replicate the key exercises right at your hotel.

Just move the furniture in your room so that you create a clear area in front of the mirror. Start your workout with the same stretching and warmup exercises and mirror training you'd do normally. Then let the clear area serve as a small ring as you shadowbox. If the ceiling is high enough, you can jump rope in the same spot. If it's not, be creative: I've jumped rope in hotel fitness rooms, at poolside, in empty conference rooms, and in hotel parking lots. After jumping rope, you might do some light roadwork within close proximity of the hotel, and then head back to your room for stomach exercises.

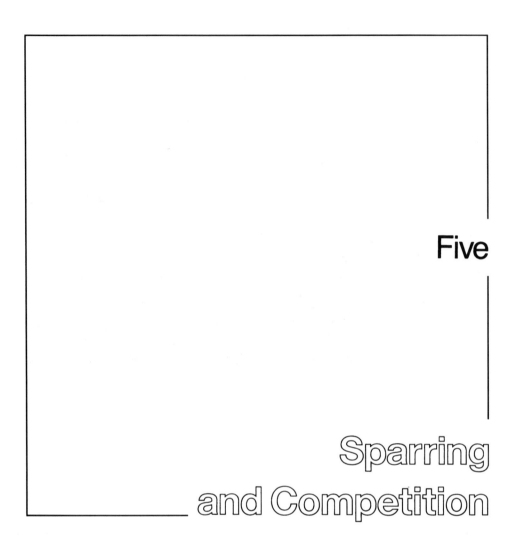

Five

Sparring
and Competition

For many white-collar boxers, the Boxer's Workout itself is enough. It gives them the fitness they want with the character they want. A growing number of white-collar boxers, however, choose to go farther and regularly partake in supervised sparring in a serious boxing gym.

Base your decision as to whether to spar on what you want to get out of boxing, and on the degree of commitment you're able to make. Sparring means you'll need to get a trainer and make regular trips to a serious boxing gym for both training and sparring sessions. (Again, you should never spar except in a boxing gym, under the supervision of your trainer.) And although sparring sessions are su-

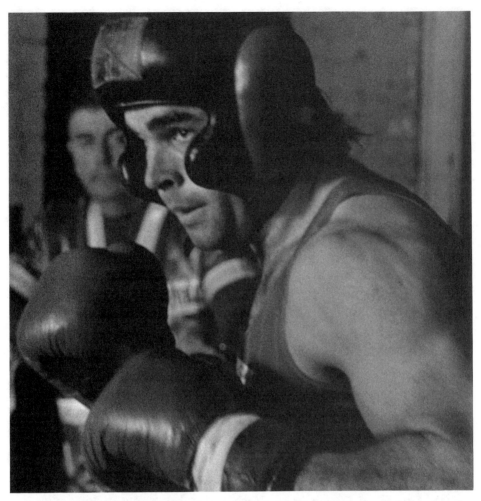

Successful sparring entails the correct application of the fundamentals under pressure.

pervised and safe, you should recognize from the beginning that you're going to get hit, at least once in a while. While many white-collar boxers wear an occasional fat lip or black eye like a badge of courage, you might not appreciate this distinction on the eve of an important meeting with a new business prospect. (It should be noted however, that your wound is more likely to serve as an interesting conversation starter than a detriment. I haven't met a client yet who isn't interested in boxing—at least on some level.

Don't consider sparring unless you've been working out at the

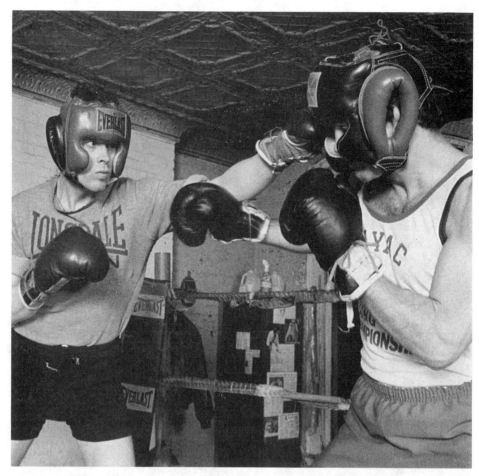

Michael Patrick Hearn, a free-lance writer and reviewer, jabs at southpaw David Foxen, an account executive with a major investment firm.

intensive level for at least eight weeks. As you step into the ring, you shouldn't even have to *think* about whether you're in good enough shape. (There's plenty to focus on without having to divert your energy to worrying about whether you're fit enough to spar in the first place.) Don't eat for at least four hours before your sparring session, and make your last meal a light one—body shots have a way of reminding you of what you had for lunch.

Successful sparring entails the correct application of the fundamentals under pressure. As you'll learn no later than your first sparring session, this can be incredibly difficult. I'd be richer than the richest arbitrageur if I had a nickel for every time I've heard a boxer outside the ring criticize the boxers in the ring, only to get into the ring himself and make the same mistakes and worse. While sparring isn't easy then, the following six guidelines will help.

1. Start by getting centered and comfortable. Breathe deeply as you step into the ring. Move around a bit before the round starts, to get a feel for the ring surface.

2. Crystallize your strategy. Using your personal boxing style as a starting point, you and your trainer will have worked up a clear battle plan before you actually step into the ring. Quickly review your strategy with your trainer before the bell rings. Remember that in general the following points hold:

- If you're boxing a (taller) boxer, you'll need to cut the ring, get inside, and then punch in combination.
- If you're boxing an infighter, jab and circle. Step in with combinations, and then step out and resume your jab-and-circle pattern. Stay out of the corners.
- If you're boxing a counterpuncher, feint and draw in order to make him lead, and then counter his lead with combinations. Beyond those basics, you should also consider what your opponent expects you to do. Without changing your basic style (you should almost always stick to your bread-and-butter), are there any new wrinkles you can introduce to confuse him?

3. Set the pace and control the action. Don't start throwing punches willy-nilly as soon as the bell rings. (Too many beginners punch themselves out in the first round.) Move behind your jab and establish the pace that benefits you, that is in keeping with your style. If your opponent is pressing the action too much for your liking, jab and move away until he punches himself out or begins to swing wildly. If he's moving too slowly, step in behind your jab and quicken the pace. Control the action. (The oldtimers call this "ring generalship.")

4. Note your opponent's tendencies and capitalize on them. Does he lower his right when he throws his left? Slip inside his jab and counter with a straight left to his chin followed by a straight right. Conversely, do you find him "waiting on" your straight right, after every jab you throw? Surprise him with a hook off your jab.

163

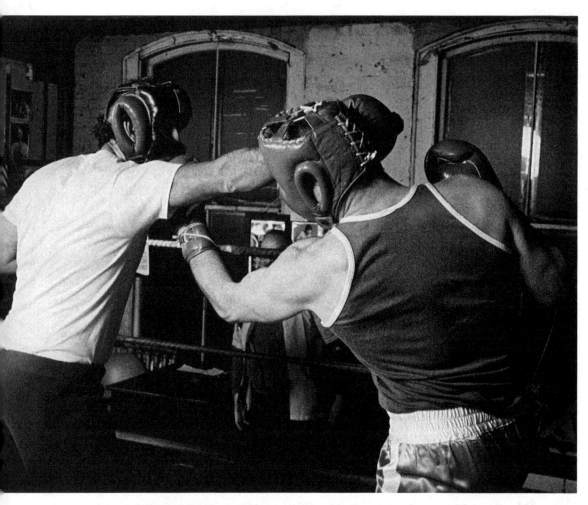

Tom Gimbel slips outside the left jab of Alan Caminiti and counters with an uppercut.

5. If you get hit, stay under control. Move away behind your jab, or step forward and clinch. Breathe deeply. Clear your head and find your center before resuming under control. Remember to keep your hands up.

6. Evaluate and plan during the "rest" minute. Breathe deeply as you listen to your trainer between rounds. He'll tell you what you're doing right and what you're doing wrong. He'll describe the tendencies he sees in your opponent. Finally, he'll tell you exactly what to do during the upcoming round. Listen to him carefully, and execute as best you can.

Above all, be patient with yourself. You'll probably find that during your first few sparring sessions you abandon a surprising amount of the technique you'd practiced so diligently. Stick with it. Like anything else, it takes time and practice to improve. And I guarantee you that you will improve. Rather than getting emotional about it, evaluate each sparring session clinically, with the help and advice of your trainer. Isolate those things you need to work on, and give them extra time during subsequent floor exercises. Similarly, give yourself credit for the things you did well, and be sure to make them an important part of your battle plan next time.

A Note on Fighting Southpaws

Many right-handed fighters cringe when they have to face a southpaw. The reason for this apprehension is that the southpaw is necessarily more familiar with fighting opposite-handed fighters than is the right-hander.

Fighting a southpaw effectively need not be mysterious, however. The key is to remember to always move toward your left, away from his power punches—that is, his straight left and left cross. If you're a boxer, jab and move toward your left. If you're an infighter, favor your left side as you work to get inside. By continually forcing the action to your left (his right), he'll be forced to deliver his power punches across his body. You'll be able to "pick up" and defense them relatively easily, and there's a good chance he'll be left off balance. Additionally, throw a greater number of straight right leads than you otherwise might, launching this punch between the southpaw's gloves. Finally, beware of the southpaw's right hook. Initially you might find it unusual to see a hook coming at you from your left side.

Afterword

Requiem
for a Boxing Gym

I appreciated the Gramercy Gym the most when it was empty. Every now and then, I'd stay behind to lock up after everyone had gone. It was usually so noisy when boxers were working out that the quiet that took over when they left was kind of special. During summer, the last rays of light would hit the lockers in the back of the gym just right, as if to illuminate the story inside each one.

On January 21, 1987, the light went out for good. At about four-fifteen that afternoon a city building inspector walked into the Gramercy and told Al Gavin that the old walkup building

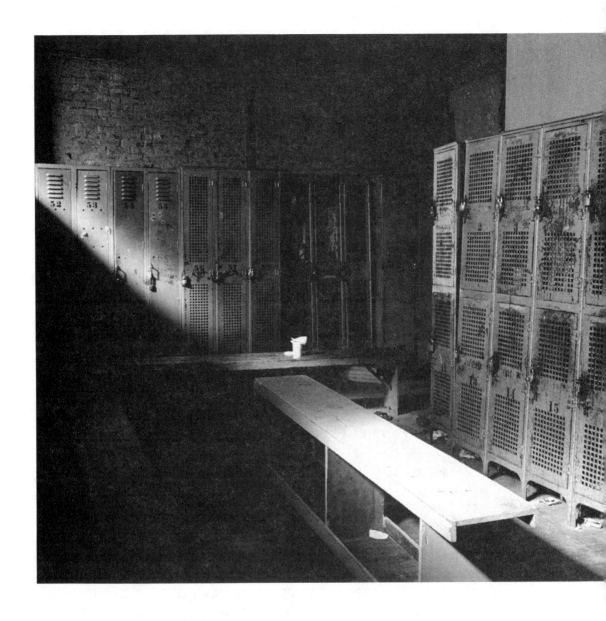

that housed the gym was being closed, ostensibly to be demolished. There had been an electrical fire in the building a few days before, and the city (which was also the landlord) had determined that it was too expensive to install the new wiring system needed to make the building safe. Al and Bob Jackson had kind of known this might be coming. The area immediately around the gym had been under redevelopment for some time (gourmet grocery stores, expensive co-op apartments, etc.). The gym building, in its downtrodden glory, was beginning to stick out like a sore thumb, and on a prime piece of real estate at that. The electrical fire gave the city a perfect excuse to do now what it was probably going to do later anyway. As he left, the inspector threw the master switch that turned off the lights.

We were all a little lost for a few days. Some of the boxers I'd worked out with for years at the Gramercy called up. We talked to each other as you do when there's a death in the family. "It's the end of an era. They just don't make 'em like that anymore," said one good friend. Another angrily said, "It was beautiful: a small, unpretentious neighborhood boxing gym. And now it's gone." As bad as I felt, I was thankful that the opportunity to write this book came along when it did. I was finishing up the manuscript just as the Gramercy closed, and I realized that the photos for the book, taken at the gym a few months earlier, would wind up being the last photos ever taken there. Over the years I'm sure they'll serve well as a kind of time capsule for those who experienced the Gramercy Gym.

A few days later Al called. "We're going to Gleason's," he said. Gleason's Boxing Gym, a much larger gym with its own rich history, had just relocated from midtown Manhattan to a huge, brand-new facility in Brooklyn Heights. Its owners had invited Al and Bob to move there and stay for as long as they wanted. Since blood runs thick between trainers and their boxers, this meant that many of the "regulars" from the Gramercy would probably be making the move to Gleason's.

I moved my gear to the spanking-new Gleason's Gym and began workouts there. The first week or so was tough. It's not that the new Gleason's wasn't a fine gym—it was and is. It offers the newest equipment (including three beautiful boxing rings) and additional facilities that we would've only dreamed of at the Gramercy. But it wasn't the *Gramercy* gym. Even though Al and Bob were there, it wasn't the same gym as the one where Floyd Patterson and José Torres trained, and Rocky Graziano before them. It wasn't the home of the ghosts of countless other boxers who struggled over the years to reach the same pinnacle those three did, only to realize in the end that they wouldn't make it. Compared to the Gramercy, the new gym didn't seem to have a soul.

Now it's the middle of March. I'm still working out at the new Gleason's and starting to feel more comfortable. I've noticed that many of the boxers from the Gramercy have indeed made the move with Bob and Al. This includes quite a few white-collar boxers who, when combined with the large number of white-collar pugilists already at Gleason's, account for a significant portion of the new gym's membership.

More important, I've noticed that everyone at the new Gleason's—pros, Golden Glovers, and white-collar boxers—is working very hard, each striving to succeed. For some, that means going after and capturing a world championship. For others, it's the simple act of taking off a business suit and throwing a punch correctly for the first time. But for everybody it means making that struggle which boxing so perfectly crystallizes; with each of us confronting that precise amount and nature of fear and anxiety which is uniquely ours, and somehow "getting through."

It's unfortunate that the Gramercy is no more. But as I observe each boxer (including me) making his individual struggle at the new gym, I'm absolutely certain that over the years it will become hallowed ground every bit as much as the Gramercy. For in the end, the struggle is what is important.

ACKNOWLEDGMENTS

Good people are hard to find. I'd like to thank the following:

First and foremost, my wife Marian; who served as my guide and critic throughout this endeavor ("Hey, Marian, how does this section sound? Does it make sense? Or should I check into Bellevue right now . . . ?"). She gave me the constant, caring, and objective support that only a loving Black Belt could provide. She helped me to stay on center.

Vincent Aiosa, outstanding photographer and devoted friend, for the innovation and craftsmanship he brought to both the planning and execution of this project. Working under the most adverse conditions (bells ringing, boxers bouncing around all over the place, trainers yelling, limited time, cramped conditions, etc.), Vince captured not just the technical aspects but the spirit of the sport. I believe that his stop-action studio shots are truly innovative for the how-to sports medium.

Al Gavin and Bob Jackson, models of what a great trainer should be; for teaching me everything I know about boxing, and for always being in my corner with their technical contributions and criticism, time, moral support, and friendship.

Tom Gimbel, an advanced student of the sweet science, for his technical criticism and help in choreographing and modeling the demonstration photographs.

The remaining white-collar boxers who were part of this book, especially the following, whose photographs appear in the book: Spenser Alpern, Alan Caminiti, Joseph Carberry, Joseph Egan, Robert Elsasser, David Foxen, Ray Ginther, James Grant, Michael

Groves, John Haran, George Haywood, Michael Patrick Hearn, Tyrone Howard, Robert Jaeckel, Ira Lieberman, Kevin McCloskey, Dr. Howard Miller, W. Gregg Porter, Martin Snow, Oliver (Jim) Sterling, and Brant Thomas.

Andrew Ferrari, my close friend and first client, who took a chance on me three years ago, and who provided support and encouragement throughout this project.

Norman Stahl, writer and friend, who several years ago encouraged me to turn my idea for a book on the kind of workout that boxers do into a proposal, and who helped me formalize the proposal.

Nancy Hogan of the Carol Mann Literary Agency, and Carol Mann, who believed in the idea and presented it to Dolphin/Doubleday Books.

Paul Bresnick, editor, who patiently helped this first-time author to shape the book, and whose support ultimately made it a reality.

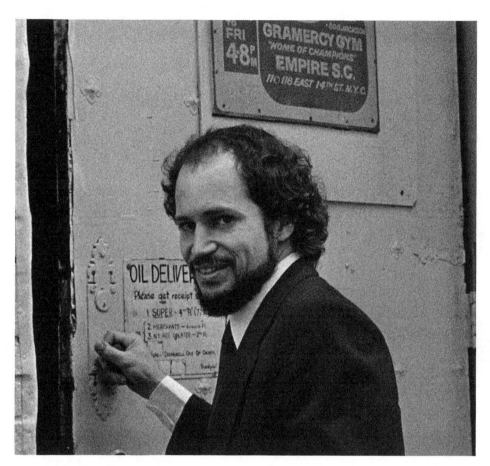

Peter DePasquale.